RECONCEIVING
MY BODY

RECONCEIVING
MY BODY

Take Two, from the Heart

Gil Hedley, Ph.D.

To order additional copies of this book, contact:
Xlibris Corporation
1-888-7-XLIBRIS
www.Xlibris.com
Orders@Xlibris.com

CONTENTS

*With gratitude to my parents, healers in their own right,
who kindly conceived my body in the first instance*

CHAPTER ONE

Coming in to Form

Why reconceive my body? Because the one I've got crackles and pops like a bowl of Rice Krispies, and the gray hairs in my beard are multiplying faster than internet stocks. Because my genes have holes in the knees. Because after my umpteenth back-outage and my last migraine headache, something else has got to give. Sometimes I've just wanted to crawl back into mama's womb and start all over again. I've at long last decided to enroll in the refresher course on how to grow a body.

I can remember hobbling about the hallways of grammar school at the ripe age of ten with a wicked backache. That was the year I had my first crisis with destiny. I must have suffered from some compulsion to know my future, because one day I put God on the spot with a prayer that only a child would pray: "God, tell me what I'm going to be when I grow up. Tell me at church on Sunday." Well, I asked for it. At the homily during mass on Sunday the priest spoke of his vocation, or call, to the priesthood, and how he had answered that call by becoming a priest. Yikes! I went home in a panic, sweating the awful truth of my future. I'm supposed to be a priest! I don't believe that that sword of Damocles hanging over me set up my youthful back troubles, but in retrospect, they make a good match.

I spent the next several years serving as an altar boy. I learned to light matches and hardly ever spilled candle wax on myself. I became comfortable working with the priests. I can remember sitting there next to one particular fellow up at the altar. During the lulls in the action, I would watch the ants crawling by our specially positioned seats. Then I would watch the priest. He was equally captivated by the ants. We were bonding over God's little creatures.

By the time I turned thirteen I sprouted some serious muscles. Eventually, I also grew to be taller than the pastor, and was unceremoniously retired from my duties. So much for the direct career path. I moved on to other projects, and let the answer to my childhood prayer drift back into the rear of my consciousness. The concept of my being a priest seemed remote. I devoted myself to the delights of building my growing body with intense enthusiasm.

In fact, I can still envision the sight of that aspiring Arnold Schwarzeneger that I was as a teen, swaggering about, chopping and stacking half a cord of wood in a morning and then popping out for a thirty mile bike ride. I can only wonder where he went. I am actually fond of saying he learned to read, then shrunk back into a normal human being. The fact is, at the time, I had an idea about what my body should look like, and then went for it. Weight training six-days a week, biking, up to a thousand sit-ups a day— I used to do four hundred push-ups in 17 minutes flat . . . the time it took to play one side of Aerosmith's "Get Your Wings." Well, I got my wings. My upper body had that flared look of a cobra about to strike. I call that the twenty-four hour lat-spread. It was all the rage in my high school locker room. My legs looked like tree trunks taken in at the waist, knee and ankle and just learning to walk. Incidentally I was in constant pain, as I was forever "ripping" my muscles, on the principle that if I "ripped" them down and then gobbled tons of protein, I would build them to even more massive proportions. So I was always waddling around on my ever-repairing legs, barely able to lift my increasingly bulging arms, all in the name of "getting big." I had occasional serious flare-ups of my earlier back problems, but I would move through them stoically and build myself up all the more. "Pain means gain" was my motto, and that was how I lived. Until I got to college.

The burden of keeping up with studies eroded the time I could devote to getting big. I guess I decided I would rather just get big inside my head than all over. Suddenly, events and choices conspired to make that possible. I got straight A's my freshman year. Well, that was a pretty good trick, I thought, but not one likely to be repeated! Early sophomore year I fell obsessively in love with a beautiful and inspiring young woman who was convinced she had giant calves. They were lovely calves, actually, but none of my sweet words or clumsy groping could convince her otherwise. Consequently, she tended towards the anorexic side of things. In her effort to make her calves disappear, she ate like a bird in flight—a very cheap date.

Her roommate at the time was bulimic. Oh, what a trio we made in the cafeteria. Keeping up with my girlfriend, I quickly lost my appetite. We would whisk through the buffet gathering a few pieces of iceberg lettuce, and the roomie would pile up some goodies, eat, and then excuse herself "for a minute." She always seemed so chipper. Since I spent so little time on eating, I had that much more time to study, and as the semester wore on I realized I was getting straight A's again. Now the pressure was on. I transferred my compulsion to get big with a compulsion to get A's. I was also deeply guilt-ridden over my sexual feelings and desires. The answer to my childhood prayer lurked within me. My girlfriend soon tired of my obsessive and controlling tendencies towards her (imagine that!) and started dating another fellow. A smart move on her part, but the sum of my guilt and shame coupled with the way I took the rejection was more than my frail being could take. I basically popped out of my body in the confusion of it all. I sort of accidentally-on-purpose dissociated myself from my body.

The "good news" was, in that state I became the ultimate study-machine. I also found all sorts of positive re-enforcement for my condition in the models of sanctity of the Catholic Church. All the Saints I'd heard about were ashamed over their sexual inclinations. I fit right in, there. And regarding the food issue, I didn't have an eating disorder. Not at all. I was *fasting*. There was certainly plenty of support for that. First, I'd skip eating one meal. I didn't even have to leave the library. Then two meals. Then a day. Then two days a week. Then a day plus a meal, once, twice. You get the picture. I no longer wanted to be big. I had a new idea. I wanted to be holy. The upshot of all this was triune. I got "holier;" I lost a considerable amount of pure, lean, hard-earned muscle mass; and I got straight A's again!

Unfortunately, my studious, dissociated and very skinny version of holiness was completely lacking in fun. I was depressed, and had no appetite. I was academically successful, but was completely dismissive of any accomplishment—humility, I called that. I was not a happy saint. One morning, after finals were over, but before I was to leave for Christmas break, I simply didn't want to get up. This was not the simple kind of not-wanting-to-get-up because the pillow is so snuggly or because the room is still spinning from last night's party. I had lost my will to live. I had been dragging my body along like some form of punishment, and I didn't want it anymore, and felt no connection to it except for loathing. That's in retrospect. I wasn't connected enough to my body at the time to understand the physical impact of dissociation. All I knew then was that I didn't want to get up. Period.

As I was lying there, however, the thought occurred to me to check my post-office box. Thank goodness. Now mind you, I had been in the habit of checking the thing several times a day, and it was empty virtually all the time. I was like Charlie Brown wanting to kick the football. However many times Lucy holds the ball, she always jerks it away at the last moment. But Charlie Brown keeps coming back for one more shot. The mailbox was my Lucy. Would it hold a letter for me this time?

I checked the box. In it, to my utter astonishment and by the actual grace of God, was a handmade Christmas card from a high-school chum. The card was a jolly drawing of Santa wishing me a merry Christmas. The word "Yup!" was written, with a dramatic arrow, pointing to the red curly hair glued to Santa's chin. It seems my redheaded (all-over) friend had drawn upon her own resources to make Santa's beard extra-realistic. I was tickled to my depths with delight, and laughed out loud. My laughter kindled hope, and though I was still in quite a pit, now I was looking up out of it rather than down into it.

Over the months that followed, hope built upon hope, and I further kindled my fires. I committed to joining friends with appetites for dinner and quit my compulsive fasting. I didn't gain much weight from that point, but I did stop losing it. I built upon my suspicion that somehow self-loathing and perpetual bodily punishment was a betrayal of the commandment to love God and neighbor *as oneself.* Then one day I paid a visit to my ex-girlfriend and she reported some significant news. It seems her roomate had admitted to both her bulimia and many associated deceptions (constant lying, stealing, etc.). She was returning items she had stolen, and asking forgiveness of her hallmates. This was a dramatically promising shift. My "ex" informed me that the roomie wanted to apologize to me as well.

I left in a deeply introspective mood, and wandered to a lovely spot to be alone and watch the sunset. As I sat, I imagined my ex's roommate coming to me to ask for my forgiveness. My response was instantaneous. *Of course I forgive you! And what for, anyway?* I returned to my room to study with some greater purpose stirring inside of me. A certain sort of Divine Logic was impressing itself upon my consciousness. The roomie had done all sorts of "wrong" things, but was undoubtedly, immediately, and entirely forgivable. That's because in the core of her being, I knew she was good. Her goodness did not depend on what she had done, but on who she was: God's good creation. She was good, because God was good in her, not on a scale of one to ten, but essentially. Then came the punch line that brought me home: the same is true for me.

The realization "*I am good*" ran through my body with the steady power of life itself. In that moment, I knew I was "back." I experienced my own re-association, having had so unceremoniously split my body off from the rest of me several months earlier.

I literally ran around excitedly announcing "I'm back" to everyone I bumped into, awkwardly explaining the provocative realization of my/our essential goodness. The discovery of gravity paled in comparison. I had discovered levity! I was on a roll. A month later I even got back together with the girlfriend. Our second go-round was short-lived, but I learned a lot. Break-up number two lacked the devastating impact of the first. I was renewed, and deeply optimistic. I sprang awake in the morning. I was charged with the knowledge of who I am: *good*.

Despite my recovery, I continued to collect my A's, took an interest in studying religion, and began to deeply explore moral questions. I took off from school for a half-year to work with service-oriented missionaries in Los Angeles, California, and Port-au-Prince, Haiti. From the example of those missionaries, I learned that unless I took constant and earnest care of my bodily needs, I could quickly end up on a cot in the ward, dying along with the folks I was supposedly there to serve. I ate my rice and beans with gusto. My faith was hearty too. I loved changing peoples' bandages at the clinic and "home for the dying." The ridiculous things I would say in my attempts to speak Creole made people in even the most desperate circumstances laugh, and I found out what a powerful healer fun can be.

I lived and worked with the Missionary of Charity brothers at their compound in *Cite Simone*, a "shantytown" of Port-au-Prince. One day a van got stuck deeply in the mud outside the compound wall within which the brothers cared for about twenty-five "street" boys. The boys called for me to help. I walked out to witness the scene of several bare-footed men struggling to push the van while its tires hopelessly spun sloppy mud out on everyone nearby. Unmovable. In what became a whirlwind of cooperation, I had the inspiration to simply get enough enthusiasm rallied for the job to just pick the darned thing up and put it on dry ground. With much grunting, counting (Un, deux, TROIS!) and adrenaline, that's exactly what we did.

Quite unpredictably, this simple experience was somehow one

of the most fulfilling of my life. As I walked from the cheers of the
scene, I was awash with feelings of exhilaration and completeness.
In retrospect, I would say I had an experience of integration and
union, both in myself (body, mind and spirit), with others (the
co-operating group of van-lifters and onlookers) and with the Divine (it almost seemed as if that van picked itself up in the final
instance!). I felt in love again, with no girlfriend in sight. At the
time, all I could put together were the basics. I feel incredibly
good; I am with the brothers in Haiti. I linked the two, and concluded I would forgo going back to college, and my entire former
life for that matter, and join the brothers. Clarity at last! It seemed
a little strange to me that the brothers weren't priests, but I figured it was close enough to the original "mandate" set out in answer to my childhood prayer.

I was elated. I can't say the same for my family. Desperate,
painful letters followed the announcement of my intentions. My
family was devastated. Lucky for me I had been intensely reading
about St. Francis of Assisi at the time. It seems Francis had also
made moves to reject his former life in favor of brotherhood in
Christ, and his family was none too happy about it either. "Christ
came to bring not peace, but the sword," I reminded myself, "and
to turn father against son and mother against daughter." Well,
sure enough, that was how things were playing out. "The one who
chooses to follow me must leave behind his family." Okay, I
thought. These are the sorts of scriptures one whips out under
such circumstances. It worked for Francis, after all. The more viru-
lent their groanings got, the more confident I became that I was
making the right decision. Such was my logic. Apparently the
scriptures were being fulfilled on the spot.

Lucky for all concerned, the story doesn't end there. Over the
course of the previous year and a half, I had been "growing accustomed" to perspective-shifting realizations, whisperings from
within, and visionary prayer experiences happening on a regular
basis. They still shook me with the force of a surprise, but I was
starting to like surprises. I was now very ripe for another big "Aha!"

After receiving communion at daily mass one morning I was over-whelmed with the very real and palpable sense that Jesus was im-mediately though invisibly present to me. I felt him. A communi-cation took place in a moment which took me the rest of the day to "translate" into words. I guess I'm still trying to translate the experience, both into words and practice. Perhaps this was a psy-chological stress reaction to family turmoil and isolation in a strange place. Maybe I had an "official" prophetic experience. Or perhaps "C," all of the above, or "D," neither. The bottom line was, by any account I had a profoundly "functional" experience.

The words *Remember Abraham* kept echoing inside of me. Abraham was the Bible hero still remembered as the "man of faith." That's because when he heard God's call to sacrifice his only son Isaac, the old whacko was actually going to go through with it. Lucky for Isaac but unlucky for a ram caught in a nearby thicket, God suggests a last minute switch, and Abraham reaps major re-wards for having followed God's call in the moment once again. The analogy hit home. Sacrifice took on a new meaning: it was about letting go, and offering. I had let go of my past by offering to join the brothers. Like Isaac, my family got the short end of the stick in that deal. But there is a "big picture," after all. Having offered to let go, I understood that like Abraham I was to receive "the sacrifice" back, and then some. More blessings than I could comprehend. I was to have my family and life commitments back, but I could never look at them the same way. They seemed more like gifts to me now, among many, and to be held more lightly. I was filled with a sense of freedom and renewed purpose. Whatever I was to do, I could always look for clues in the moment. The experience did not seem to "re-iterate" any patent necessity that I become a priest. It dawned on me that perhaps I could even marry.

What was obvious to me was that God did not require or even want a sacrifice of painful self-deprivation. Offering to let go was an act of faith, and lucky for me, I had some. But, boy, did I look stupid. A regular pancake: flip, flop. Oh well. I knew in my heart what St. Paul meant when he said he was a "fool for Christ." I figured no one would possibly "get" what had happened. The missionaries would think I was abandoning my newly recognized vocation by yielding to the pressure of my family. But I knew I was continuing to listen to the call and allowing it to blow me where it would. My family would think I had come to my (their) senses. And I really had come more fully into my senses at every level. I could actually see more clearly. I was vibrant. But the sense of propriety which guided my family's hopes and love for me were not my guiding light at this point. I felt very connected.

I returned from the trip a new creation once again. I had an unshakable surety of faith and determination to fulfill my life's vocation. My destiny was a moving target. I also found more justification for being a tad rigid in my self-disciplines. Life with the brother's had made its mark, and not too subtly. I kept my hair unfashionably short, wore the same clothes and ate the same food every day, and I slept on the floor (for the next eight years!). This episode in my life could be titled "St. Francis goes to Duke." Despite my initial attempts to reinterpret the meaning of sacrifice, I hadn't rooted out the pain-means-gain thing completely. This should not come as much of a surprise. As a small boy of five, I can remember asking my sisters if they wanted to play "crucifixion." I wanted them to pretend to nail me to the cross, etc. Such an ambitious little fellow! Who could have predicted my later aspirations from that?

Furthermore, my ambivalence towards my sexuality still ran deeply. I could accept that saints should be happy and love themselves, but I surely wasn't seeing a grand history of folks getting canonized for fully integrating their sexuality with their spirituality. I developed a relationship early senior year which placed the issue squarely in my lap, as it were. Now I really wrestled with the question of marriage. I wrestled with the girlfriend too. She was quite a sport. My family still taunts me fifteen years later that I bought her a new laundry basket for her birthday. It *was* a really nice one.

Getting married struck me as a very complex issue. It seemed that for married Catholics, the holy part of your life came when your spouse died or you got deathly but heroically ill, or otherwise quit "doing the nasty." The more secure route was to abstain from sex entirely, as in "religious life." Thus priests and nuns and the like were championed as the more complete earthly imitators of life in the heavenly kingdom. Holier than the married folk, that's for sure. On this account, in the Kingdom of God, presumably everyone is cut off from their sexuality.

Putting it this way, what I should do with my life seemed *sort of* logically obvious for me, and I started to become a self-conceived priest in the making again. Several fellows and I would periodically get together to feel out the possibility with the local vocations director. Our girlfriends were not at all fond of these meetings, dubbed by them the "Future Priests of America Club." They knew he had recently snatched an MD into his priestly lair, and feared his spell over us. He also seemed to have a decent expense account with which to woo us, and we enjoyed being courted. But I was coming to the concept on my own, and not merely by fiat.

There were, however, still some major kinks to be worked out. To be holy, I could be happy, but certainly not sexual. And if I *was* sexual, well then, I darn well ought to feel guilty (for failing my aspirations to holiness as so clearly articulated by my beloved Church and favorite saints). I was definitely finding it hard to be as alive and happy as I felt and not simultaneously have my sexual energies stirring my loins on a regular basis. Constantly, in fact. The spirit was willing but the flesh was "weak." And what with all that chronic optimism and happiness and genuine good cheer and delight, it was easy to be in love. I prayed with St. Augustine, "Lord, make me chaste . . . but not yet."

Unfortunately, I was in a state of constant guilt. I would drive wedges between me and my girlfriend with the guilt and sense of betrayal of my half-chosen vocation. I eventually became insufferable, and the relationship ended. I began to loathe and resent "having" to become a priest again, a "choice" which seemed by the logic of holiness to be compulsory if I was to get my "A" in Sanctity. That's the class that really counted for the big GPA (grade point average) of life. I was in a double bind, and these were my choices. I could either take up a second-class ticket to heaven and true sanctity on earth by getting married. Or, I could become a priest, and cut off my sexuality (i.e., die) or keep it and be forever guilty. Now there are two swell options. Which would you choose?

Graduate school. That's a good answer to such a complicated moral dilemma. The Church taught that marriage was a good vocation, calling it a Holy Sacrament. This despite the fact that it was undisputedly a second-class vocation. The aforementioned St. Augustine had even written a treatise called "The Good of Marriage" (after he had abandoned his long time lover, the mother of his son, to become a priest. Take his word for it, will you?). The church also taught that the Priesthood was a good vocation, a first-class shot at sanctity, marked by the Sacrament of Ordination. But priests are not to marry, by definition being celibate according to the current doctrines of the Roman Catholic Church.

I spent the better part of eight years in graduate school working out this issue for myself and anyone who cares to read my dissertation. I believe four people have as of this writing: three were on my committee, and the other was my mother. It's so dry you could sand wood with it. Such can be the nature of academic writing. My wife, Karen, encouraged me to write this book from my heart, rather than my head. Perhaps it will have a broader readership as a result. Who can say? During the time I spent getting an MA and a Ph.D. in Religious Ethics, I racked up a few more major realizations. After the first year, I recognized that I was a terrible tease to the priestly vocations directors of various orders who were courting me, and I wrote them all "Dear John" letters. One of them was actually named John. I had several good female friends during my Masters program, and I finally knew myself well enough to acknowledge I could never be fulfilled by becoming a priest. I wanted an honest to goodness partner for life, sexuality included.

I just knew I wanted to marry (someone!), but needed to work out the theological and moral logistics of it all first. I was primed to challenge one of my most basic self-conceptions: God wants me to be a priest; I am supposed to be a priest. I had begun to suspect after my experiences in Haiti that God didn't necessarily require me to be a priest. I could always reinterpret the answer to my childhood prayer as having been a generic invitation to listen to God's call and leave out the part about the priesthood. That kind of hair splitting was beyond my ten-year-old mind; in graduate school, it was my specialty. The second part was trickier. The belief that all the logic of holiness as I understood it, and the teachings of the Church, made the notion that I *should* be a priest a real thorn in my side. Nonetheless, I knew from my study of ethics in college that what one *should* do is not always so obvious. The *reasons* one gives for what one should or shouldn't do aren't always very good ones, and can be critiqued.

I would put it all up on the block for a serious looking over: the Church's teachings on holiness, the priesthood and marriage, as well as my own deep-seated self-image. This would be a critique of my very life. After that was covered, I figured the practical matter of finding a partner in marriage would work itself out. All this, as you might imagine, turned out to be a major and lengthy undertaking for me. Other folks fall in love in high school or college, get married and live happily ever after (or divorce, and jump right back in there), right? But no, Gilly has to master the entire history of western philosophy, marriage theology and canon law and then write a book about it before he'll do it. I put myself to the tasks of graduate studies and my motivating question with fairly ferocious intensity. My back complained more and more, and I experienced periodic total debilitations. It seems my body actually had something to say about all of this, but its language was foreign to me at this point.

In addition to admitting to myself that I wanted to be married, and in light of my back problems, I noticed a peculiar thing about the nature of graduate school. It is designed to suck you out of your body and leave you hovering over it in a realm of pure intellect. The needs of your body are both irrelevant and ignored. You cook and eat because you have to. You spend long hours in lectures, straining to listen and take notes at unspeakably uncomfortable chair/tables. Exponentially more hundreds, then thousands of hours are spent reading. You read, you get up to pee and get a drink of water, you read some more, you get up to pee and drink . . . you get the picture. You hydrate and pee only to read some more. The tables and cubicles of the library all have squared-off hard edges and the lighting is cool-white fluorescent. If you actually read everything that is assigned, you will simply read in perpetuity. Now don't get me wrong, there are certainly luxuries that come with the life of the mind. These are obvious to those who like to read! After a few years I realized that taking classes and even meeting with professors were simply distractions from reading. Later in my graduate career, I just went to the library seven days a week for five and a half months to read one author, St. Thomas Aquinas, all day long, often in Latin. To quote Bob Marley, may he rest in peace, "You think you're in heaven but you're living in hell! Oh, time will tell, yeah, time will tell."

CHAPTER TWO

Fishing for Clues

After the first year I had my masters degree, and I took a year off to fund the next stage of study. I worked, as I had in the in-between times in the past, on a garbage truck. I was into extremes. Being a "garbage man" is serious physical work. Running around and lifting trash all day long, hopping up and down from the cab of the truck in the great outdoors: I got into great shape relative to my ghostly studious state. My back only "went out" seriously once that year. I missed a week of work but slowly recovered. I rode my bike after work, renewed the relationship with the college girl-friend at a distance, and went to mass every day for spiritual refreshment. By the end of the year, I hoped she might marry me, but my hints and queries made it clear that I was, though a good fellow, still a bit of a personality-overdose to make her an appropriate life-partner. I was a bit intense. I'd have to work on that one, I realized. Time was on my side.

I returned to graduate school more connected to my body and I could see some indisputable value in that fact. I wanted to maintain the connection, and also support my back-needs while at school, so I joined the Tai Chi Tao club at the University. Tai Chi is sort of like yoga that gets up and walks around. Chinese "bird dancing," as I used to call it. Slow, intentional movements are done in groups or individually, for health, mental training and martial sport. As was my pattern, I became a fairly obsessive "Tai Chi guy." I practiced as a break from reading and took as many classes as I could. My body patterning had been incredibly rigid;

I had grown accustomed to fearing my own movement on the grounds that I might hurt my back. Tai Chi brought more movement into my life and body, and I clung to it like a lifeboat.

As I chipped away at my physical rigidity, my roommate chipped away at my dogmatism. I held church teachings as tightly as I held my back. My roomie was on the other side of a similar pattern. We would hit the lights for bed, and then start talking about theology. One by one he would challenge my beliefs, and I slowly began to loosen up around them. I can remember begging to keep just one little dogma for myself, but he was unrelenting. My big bag of dogmas got smaller and smaller until it was nearly empty. I fought for them all to the end. It was, however, incredibly refreshing to develop and cherish beliefs because I experienced their truth, and not merely because they fit my holding pattern or because I thought I was *supposed* to believe them. I also began to suspect that there was a direct correlation between the loosening up of my body from Tai Chi and the loosening up of my belief system. The two activities were mutually supporting. I wondered what my study of theology and ethics might turn into if I kept "getting into my body."

The roomie introduced me to a social work student who I later met again at church. It was love at second sight. After a few months of intense getting-to-know-each-other, it seemed I had finally met my match. We left for the summer in opposite directions, she to volunteer in Canada with mentally handicapped adults, and I for several months to a day center for people with AIDS in Oakland, California. This cracked some more of my rigidity. At the time, AIDS was still primarily a "gay plague." I was suddenly surrounded by "gay" culture, and found myself laughing constantly amidst devastating illness, much as I had in Haiti. Campy humor and innuendo kept me in stitches. One fellow, who called himself the African Queen, even proposed to me. I told him I was already engaged, thank you, and he promptly offered to marry her as well! I witnessed supportive devotion and love, for better or for worse, among men there as I had never seen it in my life. The sick were treated as beloved persons, not as victims. We discussed my study of marriage theology and ethics, and I was challenged to write something that could speak to the needs and realities of all committed couples. My dogma-bag was sounding pretty hollow at this point.

Regarding my "fiancée," as we had informally come to regard each other, I held her tightly enough to suffocate us both; daily love letters and poetry went out by the post, but the return flow gradually petered out. I ignored the signs, and not surprisingly my back went out in a big way. I awoke in pain, and couldn't get off the floor (yes, I was still sleeping on the floor!). As I lay there, Bobby McFerron's silly "Don't Worry, Be Happy!" song began doodling through my mind. I wiggled my way into the next room like a broken snake and found a collection of Berke Breathed's "Bloom County" comics. I read and giggled all day, waiting till I could move again.

By the time I returned to school in Chicago, my fiancée had decided she had found her life's calling and returned to live in Canada. Despite all of her hints, I just couldn't accept being passed over for another love, even though it wasn't a particular person. I was furious and played the victim to the hilt. I tapped into a lifetime's worth of anger and dumped it all in her direction. My beloved grandmother had died a few weeks earlier, so I was simultaneously overwhelmed with grief. Sadness and anger. I was awash with intense emotions. This was actually not a bad thing. Between the sobbing and the wall-punching, I fit right in to the crowds of people writing dissertations in the neighborhood. I figured there were more people talking out loud to themselves on the south side of Chicago than in Bellevue. This state, incidentally, lasted for two solid years. Whoever said "nice guys" can't hold a grudge! The incidences of back-outages increased in frequency, and I practiced Tai Chi all the more, at least two hours a day. It was a finger in the dike, at this point. Something else needed to move. My pelvis. It took a few more years for me to figure that one out, though. I was still too busy *thinking* about marriage.

And what a great conversation starter *that* makes for a first date. After two years the volcanoes of my pent-up emotions quieted enough for me to see through my own smoke and ash and spot a lovely woman from Tai Chi class in the library. We began seeing each other outside of class on purpose, one thing led to another, and we became a couple. She was several years older than I, her friends were married with children, she was finishing up her Ph.D. and had already been hired to teach at a University. My infantile foot-stomping suddenly seemed remote and boring relative to an actual mature adult relationship.

I helped her relocate to Florida and spent the summer there studying for qualifying exams while she settled-in to the new job. Despite the fact that I hadn't worked out all the details justifying marriage in my mind, I was forging ahead once again. I still tortured myself about issues of sexuality, but I took a huge step. I switched pictures at my little shrine. Down came the solemn and studious image of St. Dominic reading a manuscript, and up went St. Joseph bouncing the baby Jesus on his knee. I may still have been rigid, but at least I knew it. I needed a new mirror.

I sought out a local Tai Chi teacher for private lessons. He was an odd fellow who lived in a trailer park and ate nothing but oranges. He was in training to be a breathetarian, he told me, living off of the air alone. It seems he had worked himself off of everything but the state fruit. I suppose if he had lived somewhere else, artichokes could have been the final frontier. I was impressed. He was a big guy, so I reasoned he must have known what he was doing. I figured he could teach me how to feel and move my chi (the living energy force Tai Chi people like myself were concerned about). I had mastered feeling anger and sadness: now I wanted to have some fun with the pleasures of chi. He told me to take several deep breaths and hold while standing in a certain way. Then I would surely feel my chi. I went home to practice: stand, breath, hold. . . . I heard a distant thud. That thud was me, hitting the floor, passed out. My chi might have been moving, but this was dangerous stuff! Thank God for carpeting.

I eventually graduated to moving chi with my girlfriend and with several intervening steps, proposed that we marry. She said she'd think about it and we went out for the day to canoe among the crocodiles in a nearby estuary. Paddling alongside boat-length reptiles in a swampy river proved an inauspicious backdrop for reflecting on a future together. She turned me down. She couldn't quite trust some of my religious and doctrinal baggage. After a good night's sleep she recanted and asked me to marry her, but her arguments the day prior had been so convincing I turned her down! I couldn't trust my baggage yet either. We parted friends (it really is possible!) and I returned to Chicago to iron out some more of the wrinkles in my self-image.

And a funny thing happened on the way to my Ph.D. My mother got Rolfed®. I was visiting my parents for whom I was in the habit of giving accupressure massages, which I had learned in Tai Chi class. My mother's shoulder blades in the past had been immobile blocks attached with just so much cement that she could still brush her teeth. Now they moved quite freely, and I was shocked at the change. What happened? She told me she had gone to a "Rolfer" for a series of sessions and that was just one of the benefits. Her sciatica was gone too. I had had minor exposure to this work in the past. Once my arms and hands had frozen up after some long days painting tenements one weekend. A week later I was worse, with loss of function in one hand. My Tai Chi teacher sat me down with my arm outstretched on a table and dragged his elbow down it. I squealed with pain. He said he'd picked up the technique from his Rolfer. No one I wanted to meet soon. But when I got home, my problem was greatly improved. I used my other elbow to run down my own arm some more, and the next morning there was no trace of immobility or injury. In my part time office that day a co-worker complained of painful "shin-splints." I knew the cure. I dragged my elbow down his lower leg, and after letting out a yelp, he admitted as he hopped about our office that he felt dramatically better. On a third occasion, I had traded work with a friend of a friend—I gave him an accupressure massage and he gave me his "unauthorized" version of a Rolfing session. I felt like parts of me had been touched and connected that I didn't know I had, and was startled by the potent impact of educated hands.

When I learned my mother's whole-body transformation was rooted in her Rolfing experience, I was reminded of my former experiences and knew I had to learn more. Besides, my back was a disaster. I used to pray, Oh God, could you just give me another spine? And, since I was starting to see the light at the end of the tunnel of my degree program, I had already begun wondering about alternative career paths. Most of my friends wanted to be university professors in religious studies departments. I had come to Chicago because I was struggling to work out certain issues about marriage and the priesthood as already described. I had no particular goal of becoming a professor. Such are the luxuries of surviving on student loans and part time jobs. I had no practical concept of making a living other than driving garbage trucks. As it became obvious that I would eventually have to *pay* for all of this reading and writing, I grew practical. Perhaps law school?

Rolfing seemed like something I could make a living at and be of service as well. Maybe it would even help my back. Being adept at research, I researched Rolfing. The more I learned, the more I liked. Ida Rolf, Ph.D., called herself an educator, partly because she taught people about their bodies through touch and partly to protect herself from the medical "authorities." It was her intent that by "integrating bodies," she would help folks to mature as people as well. Her work was a potent support for healing. Jesus taught and healed. This seemed like a worthwhile combination to explore. Jesus and Ida and Gil: teachers and healers. I liked the idea.

The only way to really get to know about Rolfing, however, is to get Rolfed. So I started baking cookies. I had been experimenting with a recipe. With tips from friends, I perfected it and began to sell them on campus. I paid for my Rolfing series (and my rent) with Gil's Oatmeal-Sunflower Seed Cookies: They Sound Like

They're Good for You, *But They're Not*! I baked and sold fifteen thousand cookies that year. My entrepreneurial spirit was nourished, if not the local sugar and fat addicts.

After my first "official" Rolfing session, I cried on my way to the bus. Tears of joy. I could feel my spine moving as I walked. I felt like a wave. The permission I gave myself to move as a result of that session still ramifies throughout my life. I had been holding my spine like a telephone pole for many years, and now I could sway in the breeze like a live tree. I was still a bit wooden, but now I saw the potential to liquefy. I saw my Rolfer once a week for ten weeks, each session accomplishing different goals towards the larger purpose of whole-body integration. Halfway through the series, I actually asked him if he was *sure* he was *Rolfing* me, because his work was not painful. I learned it was imitation without knowledge that was painful, however accidentally helpful. I was definitely getting the real McCoy (McRolf?).

Meanwhile I feverishly outlined my dissertation. The project was titled "Marriage, A Habit of Love: A Constructive Critique of Contemporary Papal Marriage Teachings." I planned to review the major teachings of the Roman Catholic popes about marriage over the last hundred years or so. These were the most recent versions of the Church's doctrines over which I had been struggling for years. On the bright side, I would show why they at least made sense to the popes, and that they had a certain internal logic to them. Then I would show where they sort of missed the boat. Just because something makes sense to you, doesn't mean it does to anyone else. Also just because an authority teaches something, that doesn't mean the teaching holds together very well or is even effective. Maybe the reason I was so deeply confused by the Church teachings on marriage was because they simply didn't make good sense! I wanted to show, word for word, exactly what was confused in the popes' teachings on marriage. Then I wanted to say something about marriage that made more sense. Once I had a detailed outline of the whole project, with the basic arguments made, I stuffed it all in a folder about the way a squirrel buries acorns for winter. I would come back to it when I was ready. My tenth Rolfing session was coming up and I was on my way to Colorado for a pre-training at the Rolf Institute of Structural Integration in Boulder.

Throughout my Rolfing sessions my body awareness increased tremendously. I was being led on a detailed tour of my body, with repeated invitations to listen to it carefully, feel it thoroughly. I could see changes of my shape in the mirror from one session to the next, even from the start of one session to the end. More of me moved. When I got home from session ten, though, I hit a wall. Or rather the floor. My back "went out" as it hadn't in months. I became as instantly depressed and angry as I had been jubilant. Here I was, all excited about going to the Rolf Institute in a week, and I couldn't even get off the floor. My body felt as if there were a knife in my spine between the shoulder blades while a bowling ball was simultaneously hanging off my forehead by a chain. Un-fortunately, this situation was commonplace for me, but through-out my Rolfing series I had convinced myself it would never hap-pen again. I had gone to a chiropractor in the past without much luck. A year earlier in utmost desperation I had crawled to a medi-cal doctor whose idea of helping me amounted to mocking the chiropractor and mistaking the curvature of my spine for a tumor. Tai Chi was my mainstay, but in Rolfing I was looking for Salva-tion.

The good news was that the pre-training in Colorado included daily massage exchanges. Although I showed up looking like a recently Rolfed old man, the daily touch regime of the training was exactly what I needed. I recovered faster than usual, and felt like a fish in water in the classes. This was nothing like college or graduate school courses where students sit taking notes from pro-fessors at podiums from neatly evened rows of chairs. Here we flopped on the floor or each other, while the teacher comically pranced about showing how muscles and movements related, pe-riodically whipping off this or that article of clothing to show us exactly what he meant. In a seminar in graduate school, the model for interaction between students was war: students waging intellectual battles with each other or the professors, ever struggling to win a point and be perceived as right or smarter than the loser. Victories under those conditions tend to be sour ones at best, always coming at the expense of someone else. At the Institute, we shared a common goal of learning about our bodies, and we helped each other to do so. We were not in competition: we were in community. I had had a teacher in college who spent his career forming communities out of classrooms. He truly bucked the trend of intellectual one-upmanship. Here we added our bodies to that formula, and I loved it even more. I got an inkling of how I might enjoy teaching as well.

After five intense, full time weeks I gained the skills to give a decent massage. I also left with five months worth of home-study assignments in massage, physiology, anatomy, kinesiology and psychology. So much for the dissertation. I baked cookies, gave bargain massages, and completed the pre-training course requirements before returning in May for another week of coursework, finals and an interview to be admitted to the next step of training to become a Rolfer. While my back flared up periodically, the intensity of the problem diminished and the episodes didn't last as long. I took this as a good sign, while regretting the imperfection. I loved using my skilled hands to help people and my talent developed in proportion to my growing experience. My Rolfer recommended I see a woman for ongoing support of my bodily changes, and I did, every other week for the following year and a half. She was an Occupational Therapist who had begun to dabble with a private practice doing hands-on work. With her work I kept my hopes up that I could heal my back problems, and I thrived with her help.

Much to my delight I passed the pre-training and was accepted into the program to become a Rolfer. My professors were curious and bemused. What's Hedley gotten into now? As it turned out, several faculty suffered chronic back problems as well. Tenure obviously didn't solve all of life's worries. I hadn't quite admitted to them, or perhaps even to myself, that I would not follow in their footsteps to a career at the podium. I was certain, however, that the only way to resolve my back problems was to understand them better. I had no plans to suffer endless dull pain, periodically excruciating, for the rest of my life.

Nor did I have any plans to go to Europe, but life is full of surprises. My dear cousin was graduating from college. His folks wanted to send him to Europe with a companion, and I was the lucky chosen one. They talked my folks into footing my half of the bill, and off we went soon after my return from Colorado. We were perfect travelling companions. A couple of quiet, well mannered guys going to mass at every church we stumbled upon. At fifty dollars a day, we couldn't get into too much trouble. In fact, we could barely eat, after paying for accommodations, museum fees and souvenirs for friends and family. We learned to stretch baguettes, brie and salami like Jesus could loaves and fish. The experience we most longed for was to be accosted by gypsy children. Everyone had warned us of the marauding bands of gypsy children in Rome. We went prepared. Our money and passports were belted inside our shirts. I even sewed secret pockets into my pants. Our joy was complete when a sweet little girl offered to sell us a newspaper while her accomplices surrounded us, rifling through our empty pockets before we could shoo them away.

Since this happened three days into the trip, we wondered what peaks were left to scale. Standing outside a large piazza with some great big buildings in Rome, we summoned an overdressed fellow with our broken Italian to tell us what we were looking at. We realized the power of having a tour guide when he told us it was St. Peter's Basilica and Vatican City. The cause for his costume was that he was a member of the Swiss Guard. We had stumbled upon the epicenter of all of the teachings I had been struggling with my whole life. We found an office where you could get passes for an audience with the pope. I fully expected to shake his hand and eat wine and cheese with a few nuns or something. I spent the day leading up to our personal meeting constructing a brilliant and windy sentence in Latin which would kindly convey the sentiment of my dissertation to his holiness. In the last year I had already had several dreams of meeting the pope and speaking to him about my ideas on marriage. He wasn't the slightest bit interested! Now I would meet him for real. Perhaps he'd even want to read my dissertation some day!

Unfortunately, ten thousand other people from all over the world also held passes to the audience. We were ushered to the very rear of an enormous auditorium to sit with the other Americans. Do they always stick the Americans in the back, we wondered? They wheeled the Pope out in a sort of throne-mobile to the center of a stage where he deftly greeted the crowd in innumerable languages. Then he received endless greetings from various groups of pilgrims. He would sort of raise one hand, elbow remaining at rest, for a children's group cheer. For a rendition of a hymn from a throng of travelling nuns, both hands might lift off in exceeding approval. We began to suspect, from our great distance, that we beheld only a motorized cardboard cut-out and made for the door. The Swiss Guard made it clear that *nobody* checks out early on the pope. We were promptly returned to our seats. There we made further observational notes on what purgatory would be like for us. I never got to deliver my sentence.

Despite the history, artistic and architectural marvels of Rome, we felt a bit of a spiritual vacuum there, which wasn't filled until we arrived in Assisi, home to St. Francis, whose example I had so admired. I adored St. Francis, although I had grown to suspect something was "off" in his example the more I had developed my connection with my own body through Tai Chi, massage and Rolfing. Francis tormented his body as if he were battling a plague. The rigors of fasting and his various ascetic practices left him bedraggled, blind and on his deathbed at about forty years of age. In his parting words, he actually apologized to "Brother Ass," his "pet" name for his body, admitting that perhaps he had been a little too rough on him. In college, as I recounted, I found this type of "spiritual disposition" towards my body attractive. Lucky for me, I decided to make friends with Brother Ass after all, rather than to kill him with all that holiness.

So I did Tai Chi on spots where I imagined Francis might have prayed. The chapel of the San Daminiano cross, before which Francis heard Christ speak, was open for visiting. We sat within the room for about a half an hour. When we left, we could barely speak, but both agreed to having felt an extraordinary movement within that place. It felt as if the Holy Spirit was literally blowing around the room. We must have left there with a healthy glow, as two spirited young Italian women began following us around the town. They practically begged us to let them join us in our accommodations, but all that praying had left us clueless to that sort of "opportunity," even as it knocked. Someone has to be home to open the door.

The Italians did seem to have an intense relationship with the body that left me wondering. There is a certain robust quality of physical interaction which I as an American couldn't help but notice. Every park bench seemed host to some young couple groping each other. Sculptures and paintings were full of passion detailing agonies and ecstasies of bodily form. And church after church housed some saint or another's body, in whole or in part, on display for public veneration. In Sienna, we saw St. Catherine's holy head on display. The crowd was a bit much for me to get too close, so I settled to hang out with her thumb, which was hopefully displayed on a spike in a glass case off to the side of the "head annex," like some bizarre sort of partial hitchhiker. Holiness comes at a price to the body on this account, dead or alive. If there's anything left of it after the Saint is done with it, adoring fans will rip it to pieces for the local relic collection.

After Italy, we headed for the beach at Nice on the Mediterranean coast of France. Here women were topless and beyond. For a couple of church-hopping Americans, we barely new what to do with ourselves while sunning. In the U.S. of A., if a woman accidentally flashed a breast I had always assumed the polite thing would be to turn away till matters were undercover again. Here, nothing ever went undercover. I spent the day reading Milton's *Paradise Lost* on the stony beach, fishing for clues. Two rainy days later we popped down again to the now empty beach before catching our train. Two young woman (had they followed us from Italy?) nearby were eyeing the water and I teasingly goaded them to go in. To our utter astonishment, they stripped naked in a moment and made for the water squealing French exclamations all the way. I didn't have time to ponder the sheer joy and delight of their action. I dove straight for the chilled blue waters myself just to hide my embarrassment. In the days that followed in Paris I couldn't help but wonder if all of those nice French ladies with their poodles on the subway would just as soon be frolicking naked on the beach. The thought that shame for my own body could be outstripped by exhilaration and pleasure was a novel one for me. Viva la France!

Faced with the choice of train hopping our way to Hungary or Yugoslavia, we decided for pilgrimage over goulash. Medjugorje was a little town in Bosnia Herzagovina where there had been daily apparitions of the Virgin Mary reported for ten years running. We were determined to get some action, or at least see what the fuss was about. It took us two days on a very crowded train to get there. We were convinced half of the luggage racks on board were filled with guns and ammunition. We hadn't heard the travel advisories warning Americans to stay away. Our cabinmates smoked like chimneys, and the chain-smoking trainmen seemed unconcerned to enforce the no-smoking signs. We doled out unanticipated gratuities to armed fellows at the border in US cash. The signs were in the Cyrillic alphabet. This didn't look like Kansas anymore. Fortunately, by mastering about six words in Serbo-Croation, and making up the rest in French, we made friends fast. Soon our new pals were passing us little bottles of vodka at 8 o'clock in the morning. We were like chicks under mama's wings.

Nothing could have prepared me for my experience on that little pilgrimage. For four days we sat through three-hour long masses said by the local priests, who had turned the good fortune of the local apparition into an opportunity for some heavy-duty preaching. We hiked about the little town and visited the visionaries, who would come out of their homes at appointed times to greet the crowds and report on Mary's latest messages. Pray for peace was the main theme. It was more timely a message than we ever imagined, given that the borders closed, promptly followed by all-out war a week after we left. Fasting twice a week on bread and water was the encouraged discipline to accompany the prayers. Not a bad preparation for the ensuing shortages, come to think of it.

What with all of that praying and preaching and such, I inevitably succumbed to pangs of conscience. I had never much liked the concept or experience of "going to confession," but with fifteen little booths set up outside the church for the flocks of guilt-ridden pilgrims, I couldn't resist. I entered the little confessional and greeted a skinny, pointy, grey-bearded and brown robed old Franciscan priest who had clearly been at this for a while. As I began to make my "confession," I soon realized the little fellow wasn't quite following my train of thought. It seems we didn't see quite eye to eye on what was the crux of the problem. So, I sort of launched into a lecture, as graduate students do, on some historical and theoretical background to our "discussion," with a bit of commentary on the history of the Franciscan Order to boot. As I proceeded, I could see he didn't want to hear this. Holding his baggy brown sleeved hands over his ears, vigorously shaking his head and shouting "no! no! no!" were my main clues. Finally getting a word in edgewise, the priest dutifully looked me in the eye, pronounced me a "heretic," and informed me succinctly that *he* couldn't forgive me, the *church* couldn't forgive me, and *God* couldn't forgive me. I figured that pretty much summed things up from his side of the aisle, so I stuck my hand out, gave him a firm handshake, and thanked him sincerely for our little "visit."

I walked out of that booth feeling ten feet tall. It was the very first time in my twenty-eight years that I felt truly exhilarated after "confession." I couldn't wait to tell my cousin, and we skipped mass for a long hike to chat. In the course of a few minutes, I felt like I had finally become an adult in spiritual practice. Years of anxiety lifted. I had come to a place of true revelation, however back-asswards I had gotten to it. I understood with crystalline clarity that I alone was responsible for my own actions, whatever anyone thought of them. And in my willingness to take responsibility for myself, I found real freedom. I was not a victim: not of my own faults, nor my personal history, nor the church's teachings, nor my achy body. I did not need the kind of "forgiveness" withheld moments before. I did not need approval or disapproval from outside of my own responsible self. I marveled over how it took the little brown priest's admonishments to realize I could be so free.

CHAPTER THREE

Altered States

Contraction follows expansion eventually as a natural law. Despite the breadth of the immediate revelation, I got predictably neurotic with the fasting stuff promoted around the apparitions. It wasn't long lasting though, and I eventually dropped those disciplines. And although I remained a daily mass attendee back in Chicago, I stopped taking communion, being a heretic and all. A friend noticed my quirky behavior and helped me work it out. He taught adult converts regularly, and pointed out that new members of the Church consent to "all of the truths the Church teaches," and not that everything the Church teaches is true! I realized I could indeed be an adult in my faith and not be de-facto excluded from the Church.

After our pilgrimage, we packed our rosary beads, hopped a train, and shopped for cookoo clocks in Bavaria. We drank dark beers at the Hoffbrau House and ate monster pretzels in the shadow of the oompah-band. I did Tai Chi among the naked family picnickers at the English Gardens in Munich. I was trying to get used to that. I returned to Chicago after the trip refreshed and excited to undertake the final leg of my graduate studies.

That's where I *actually* met the pope. The first thing I did in preparation for writing was read a couple of thousand pages worth of John Paul II's teachings on marriage and family, just to get a feel for the current state-of-the-art. At least no one could say I didn't take this stuff seriously. Maybe that was the root of the problem! At least the popes and I were operating from similar states of ignorance. None of us had been married. I read, wrote, read and wrote for eleven months, until I had successfully completed a two hundred and fifty-page-long argument. I vividly remember typing the last period on the last sentence of the last paragraph. I sprang from my desk, jumping all around the room with the thrill of knowing the task upon which I had set myself seven years earlier was complete. The actual graduation did not compare. My professors were happily surprised by my work. Perhaps all of my extracurricular activities sowed seeds of doubt regarding my ability to see the project through. For my part, I felt that the Tai Chi, the massage, the Rolfing, the cookies, the travel, and last but not least, the girlfriend, all provided integrity and depth to my academic research.

Somewhere before leaving for Europe I had begun a new relationship with a friend from school. The previous relationship had ended, despite the flurry of proposals, due to apparently irreconcilable religious differences. I felt I would be on safer ground to pursue a relationship for the long run with a Catholic woman. I am remembering now a former roommate's poster, with the quote, "A ship in a harbor is safe, but that is not what ships are built for." Although we shared much common ground, we seemed, however unintentionally, to fan the flames of each other's insecurities to the maximum. My body spoke to me loud and clear. Although I did Tai Chi a couple of hours a day, and got bodywork every other week, I endured virtually constant gnawing pain that year. All of my self-help efforts seemed to do little more than postpone what seemed my early and inevitable physical decline. I read scriptures and metaphysical "new age" literature voraciously, in hopes of "curing" myself. I saw a psychotherapist (not the first one, mind you!). I prayed harder for a new spine.

There actually came a point where I endured what, for lack of a better term, I refer to as a "mystical agony." I was sweeping the Coffee Shop after closing, a part-time job I had been doing for years, and playing tunes from the Irish band "U-2" for company. I was in the habit of serenading my after-hours friends in the building with my sing-alongs after passing out the leftover doughnuts. But this day turned into a sob-along somehow. I slowly became immobilized and began to weep with a deep grief. My mind began to flash on the suffering of others. I saw the faces of the local street-dwellers in my neighborhood. I remembered my father and his brothers, and felt as if I knew in the most clearly resonant way the pain they had endured, and I understood why they dealt with it the way they had. I experienced strange happenings with my body. My arms seemed to raise from my sides without intention and my fingers and hands took up various postures as these and other images of suffering flashed across the screen of my mind, while I continued to sob over it all.

In the middle of this scene, my girlfriend popped in to say "hi!" The poor woman didn't know what to make of me, and neither did I. She offered to call a buddy of mine (the dogma-crusher!) for support, but I shook my head no. Despite the strangeness of the circumstances, I was simultaneously feeling quite good. My back pain cleared noticeably. My body felt like it was opened up somehow. And with that came the clear insight that the relationship with the girlfriend somehow was not meant to continue. The future wouldn't place us together as I had hoped and imagined, despite our difficulties.

The whole scene went on for some time, but eventually came to a close, and upon returning to a more normal state I finished sweeping. Before enlightenment, chop wood, carry water. After enlightenment, chop wood, carry water. I went over to my girlfriend's apartment to talk afterwards. My body had had its say. Now my mind entered into the formula. Frankly, I was tired of major revelations. I just wanted to have a nice life, write a dissertation, have a girlfriend, get married, and live happily ever after. All of this empathy with the pain-of-my-forefathers business was just a bit much for me to take. And to boot, if I wasn't supposed to be with her, what were my options? The desert? A monastery? Guys? She was a perfectly good person with a kind heart, we had a lot in common, she had a great sense of humor, she was smart, she was cute, she was Catholic. She was plenty, and I basically decided that I was not about to be bullied around by some damned mystical agony weird emotional body-event thing. I chose to ignore it.

Expansion, contraction. As much as my back opened, it closed as if a two-by-four had been slapped between my shoulder blades. We struggled along in an increasingly atrophied version of the relationship for another eight months or so, variously punctuated with joys and hurts. What intimacy the relationship had held in its origins shriveled. With the deposition of St. Dominic for St. Joseph, and my ejection from the confessional, I had moved past my guilt-ridden experience and perceptions around my sexuality in large measure. This didn't help us as a "couple," I'm afraid. There was enough judgment flowing between the two of us to sink even a sturdy ship, in the harbor or out.

I devoted myself to my dissertation, working out in my own mind what a marriage should be, even while the relationship slowly failed. I studied and wrote in detail about the popes' understanding of marriage. There was a general agreement in the Church's teachings that marriage was "an indissoluble bond." The consent of the partners to marry was sort of a legal-spiritual super-glue. If the couple was sober in the moment and spoke their consent before a priest, there was virtually no getting that thing apart. The popes' version of marriage was a "legal thing." Marriage was a third "entity" distinct from the partners, which came into existence through consent and could be dissolved by death alone. It was no wonder why they didn't recommend it so highly.

For the popes, the relationship of the spouses frankly had nothing to do with the marriage, odd as that may seem. Oh, they waxed evermore eloquently about the love of the spouses and all over the course of the century. But when push came to shove, those two people, their children, their bodies, their personalities and their own spiritual growth and knowledge was irrelevant to the existence and state of the "marriage" as they understood it.

The moral teachings of the popes about marriage were based

on an abstract concept, rather than the actual people in the relationship. The popes consequently didn't hesitate to lay out "absolute" moral laws regarding married folks who have the most "unabsolute" and ever-changing experiences and life circumstances. The papal teachings disregarded even the possibility of divorce, because "the marriage bond" can't be dissolved. A Catholic person legally divorced due to say, desertion, and happily remarried would be considered an adulterer so long as the first spouse was alive. Yet the popes could also invent a legal concept like "annulment," where a marriage of twenty years bearing three children could be declared never to have existed. Perhaps the original consent of the spouses was shown not to count for one reason or another. Both of these positions make perfect sense if marriage is essentially a legal entity rather than the real-time relationship of the spouses. But if marriage is conceived as a human relationship, the teachings of the popes can seem strange at the very least.

Without going into all of the gory details of the papal teachings, I will share one of the most powerful lessons I learned from my research. That is, how you conceive of something has everything to do with how you *behave* with respect to that something. Feel free to re-read that sentence a couple of times! By example, if I imagine Jesus to be my friend or brother, chances are that my prayer life will be full of casual repartee and warm conversations with Jesus. But if I primarily hold for myself the image of Christ the King, Lord and Redeemer of the Universe, I'm probably going to be doing a lot more bowing and kneeling and prostrating myself before the Almighty One. Casual conversation might seem inappropriate, or even a dishonor.

As for marriage, if I conceive it to be a habit of love, I'll probably have quite a different relationship than if my marriage is an indissoluble bond. Some would say that if you can't get out of it (the indissoluble bond), then you'll stick with it and make it work. Maybe. Perhaps the indissoluble bond is just an excuse to do nothing at all towards the development of the relationship: "we 'got married' thirty years ago, and Harry still acts like I'm his mother."

Or worse, "since you can't divorce me, I will treat you like crap without risk or penalty."

If marriage is a habit of love, different demands are implied. For instance, a habit is built up by practice over time. Practice loving acts towards each other over and over again and your marriage will become a habit of love. If you don't practice, the habit will never really form in the first place. A habit once formed can also dissolve into nothing at all if practice is neglected. If you practice the opposite, picking on each other and baiting each other and bringing out the worst in each other constantly, then your marriage may be a habit, but a vicious habit. That is the kind of habit that should be broken, or transformed if the partners are willing. This conception of marriage doesn't place any meritorious value in "sticking out" a relationship which is vicious, or dead. How many people move around in a "shared" space while the corpse of the relationship lies buried in the closet for twenty years in an album marked "Our Wedding"? A marriage will be a habit of love when two people commit to it being so and act responsibly towards the practice of loving marriage. It takes two people, in a relationship, marrying each other, becoming one, loving, over and over again.

I didn't even have to get married to figure that out. And as an adult in my faith, I no longer required an authority to give me assurance that marriage was "holy enough." I had reconceived marriage in a way that made its holiness a function of the love of the spouses, rather than the definitions of the Church. I was still fairly clueless regarding the power which reconceiving my body might hold for me. But in the same way that my various relationships with women had helped me to reconceive marriage (even if not to them!), my various trainings were giving me a base of experience from which I could reconceive my body. The stork was on its way, and I didn't even know it.

Despite my joy over completing the dissertation, the relationship ground down to a painful finish. I thought back to my "mystical agony." My body had spoken in the loudest manner and I had refused to listen. Perhaps I would pay closer attention in the future. I sold off my furniture and bookcases as I prepared to move from Chicago's south side. I boxed up my books (I have *a lot* of books; they are still in the same boxes six and a half years later) and shipped them to my folks' house in New Jersey. I had concluded a huge chapter in my life, and felt fairly well exhilarated. Some years earlier I had been whining inside my head about being a graduate student, and proclaimed my half-willing martyrdom: "God, fine. If *you* want me to go through with this graduate school business and dissertation grind, I'll get you the degree." Quick as a lightening bolt I heard a reply from within, "*You* need it!" My ego took a deep breath. Once again no arduous and painful sacrifice was necessary. This was for me. And that's how it felt as I finished. Whatever contribution I may have made to the academic discipline of religious ethics paled in comparison to the deep convictions I had established in myself over the past seven years.

I hadn't just been researching ideas about marriage, either. My voracious curiosity had turned upon "the body" with the same intensity with which I had explored the Church teachings. I was reading avidly into this second field even as I was writing in the first one. I have long been fond of telling myself that I may be obsessive, but at least I manage to obsess about interesting things. I read all eight of Carlos Casteneda's books relating his bizzarre experiences under the instruction of a mysterious Yaqui Indian medicine man. Whether or not the stories were true, I couldn't say. It actually didn't matter to me. Rather, I thrilled to the basic process which Carlos endured. His world of thoughts, beliefs and fixed notions about "physical reality" were challenged, debased and turned upside down. I wanted that for myself. My way of looking at things up until that point hadn't exactly taken the world by storm. Why not try something else?

I read Barbara Brennan's *Hands of Light*. Here was a lady, a former research scientist at that, who claimed she could see an aura of light around people and interpret their relative health accordingly. Not only that, but she apparently taught others to do the same. She saw things people couldn't normally see, heard things others couldn't normally hear, and felt things others couldn't typically feel. For all intents and purposes, she sounded like a clear-cut case for a mental institution. The difference, on her own account, was that she had developed the skill of turning the flow of extrasensory information on and off at will. The folks in the institutions are often just overloaded with information they are unable to process, and break down accordingly.

I had "heard" a thing or two myself, as mentioned. In fact, after I got back from Europe, I felt like I had more than a companion or two traipsing about with me, offering advice about this and that. For instance, I had actually bought a beautiful hand knit wool sweater in Yugoslavia to give to a pal back in Chicago. She never got it. I was having breakfast one morning and saw out the window a man rooting through the dumpster in the alley behind the house I shared with fourteen other students (that's a whole other book). Clear as a bell, I heard one of those voices within announce, "Give him the sweater." I protested of course, but promptly got the sweater, put it in a bag, went out to the alley, and gave it to the fellow. I knew how to take orders. My father was a born manager. The man was a sorry sight, and I can't honestly say I felt the sweater would improve his lot much. I went back into the house, and thought what he could really use is a whole outfit. I scrambled through my closet quickly and ran back out to find him, but he was nowhere to be found. I ran up and down the nearby streets and alleys, and returned to the house huffing, puffing and confused, with an armload of undelivered duds. Where did he go? How quick can you sell a sweater in this neighborhood? Had I entertained an angel unaware? Could the angel have at least given the sweater back since angels probably don't actually need sweaters? After a couple of months like that, I finally told the unseen advice givers to bugger off. I just couldn't tell if they were training me for something, or simply distracting me from my "real world." Such are the decisions one makes at times.

Barbara Brennan's book at least offered me some categories

with which to ponder such experiences. I read about "lucid dreaming" and "out-of-body" experiences as well. Lucid dreaming is the phenomenon where you "wake-up" to your conscious state of mind while your body is still asleep. That is, you become "lucid," or clear thinking, in your dream. I talked about it with freinds, and it turns out several folks I knew had experienced the phenomenon accidentally, or even regularly. One friend told me when he "woke up" in his dreams, knowing himself to be invincible, he would drive dream cars into trees or over cliffs, just for the fun of it. A sort of demolition derby on the astral plane. It turned out my girlfriend was an extremely proficient lucid dreamer. She dreamt lucidly on a regular basis. She would have a nightmare and turn it into a party. Or a bad guy would chase her and she would turn him into a benign creature. Once she said it just didn't work, and the bad guy kept after her. That was a *really* scary dream.

I became determined to become a lucid dreamer too. First, I started writing down dream fragments, then whole dreams, then multiple dreams each night. It doesn't do you any good to have a lucid dream if you can't remember it when you wake up! Castenada's teacher had recommended looking at your hands a lot in the daytime, and then trying to see your hands in a dream as a signal to wake up. That didn't get me anywhere. Another book suggested to ask yourself in the day over and over again, "Am I dreaming?" I tried that: Am I dreaming? No. Am I dreaming? No. . . . Sure enough, in a dream I found myself asking the same question, "Am I dreaming?" Unfortunately, I had trained myself to give only one answer, "No," and I went right on dreaming!

I decided to pick out something common in my dreams that *only happened* when I was dreaming. I picked flying. I often had flying dreams, which I loved, but never actually flew during my waking hours, oddly. And virtually every time I dreamt I was flying, I would always think in the dream, "Wow, I'm finally *really* flying, how cool!" Then I would wake happy that I flew and disappointed once again that it was "only a dream." I set up the question this way. If I ever found myself flying, I would at that point raise the question, "Am I dreaming?" Before long, in a dream, I was flying. And sure enough, I asked myself as if on cue, "Am I dreaming?" Immediately I knew the answer. *Of course* I'm not dreaming—I'm *flying*! I flew over to a rooftop and discussed the matter with a bunch of other flying people, and everyone agreed we weren't dreaming, we were flying. I knew I was getting close when I woke up from that one. I changed the format once more, repeating to myself over and over again, "If I am flying, I must be dreaming." I didn't leave any room for arguments from my very gullible dream-mind. When I found myself flying, I repeated the phrase, and bam! I was "awake" in my normal (?) state of daytime consciousness, aware that my body was asleep and that I could control the course of my dream. I immediately decided to fly to outer space. I stretched out my arms like superman and shot like a rocket amidst the stars. The view was extraordinary without city lights obscuring the galaxy. But after just a few moments of lucidity, I was back to plain old dreaming again.

Waking up and *staying awake* turned out to be entirely different problems. I was happy with my accomplishment and hungry for more. Staying awake turned out to be a matter of concentration skill. I needed to be able to focus intently to maintain the lucid state in the dream. I began staring at objects intently during the day, pondering every aspect of dimension and color of a leaf, noticing the details of pattern on someone's sweater, so that I could see those details and remember them with my eyes closed as well as open. Now when I became lucid in a dream, I would immediately fly to something and stare at it, focused on details as I had been practicing in my day-waking state. I managed to have lucid dreams using that technique that lasted half an hour. This was a really fun sport, despite the training and effort.

Depending on who you read, out-of-body experiences are one of two things. Some lucid dreamers consider the out-of-body experience to be just a kind of half-baked lucid dream, because you think you have moved your consciousness out of your body when you are really just dreaming you have. But avid proponents of out-of-body experiences say these are even *cooler* than plain old lucid dreams because you can actually move your consciousness about in the "real-time" "real world" while your body hangs out in the bed sleeping. It seems even the escoteric disciplines have their politics and one-upmanship. I had to find out for myself.

One night I became lucid while dreaming, and decided now was as good a time as any to try for an out-of-body experience. I basically rolled out of my body with a static electricity sort of whoosh. It was a feeling I recognized from other dreams, where I had passed my body through walls and such: buzzzzzappp. I began floating up to the ceiling of the room, and looked down below to see my tee-shirted body sleeping next to my girlfriend. She sneezed. I shot back into my body like a bolt of lightning and immediately awoke, blown away by the intense "reality" and clarity of the experience. The transition from awake-with-sleeping-body to awake-with-awake-body was just a moment of darkness. Based on the one experience, I couldn't settle the debate in the literature between the lucid dreamers and the out-of-body practioners, but I learned one thing for sure. I needed to get some plain old sleep. I really didn't know what to do with myself out-of-body but float like some sort of graduate-student ghost. I hadn't really established a clear intent. I also realized that my nighttime dreams or illusions were not the ones I needed to wake up from. It was plain old daytime reality that I found myself frequently "sleeping" through. I wanted to wake up from the dream of everyday reality. I'm still working on that one. I'll keep you posted.

In addition to this kind of reading, I was delving a bit into "plain old science" as well. My pre-training at the Rolf Institute had rekindled a long put-off interest in anatomy and biology. In high school, our teacher took notice that a buddy and I were particularly thrilled by our rat dissection, and she offered us a cat to do after school. I loved doing dissection. I was amazed by those incredible innards. Everything fit together so perfectly. Who made that thing? What a great idea! My senior year biology teacher took us to a gross anatomy laboratory in New York City for a class trip.

Our tour guide was a podiatry student who was clearly modelling himself on John Belushi of "Animal House" fame. It was late in the year and the tops of the cadavers had been worked on and sent off to some dental school. Podiatrists saved the best for last. There were bags of human feet on shelves in the lab. On the opened tables were hemi-pelvises and legs, partially dissected. With all sorts of macabre humor, we were introduced to these human remains. He showed us how the toes would wiggle if you pulled a certain tendon. The whole thing was fascinating and disturbing at the same time. I lost my taste for chicken on the spot.

I had no idea of the depth with which the experience impressed me. Seeds were planted. I now know from much experience that first visits with cadavers easily provoke altered states. The kind of things you say to a person under those conditions can create lasting impressions. To test this theory, ask around. Not many people forget the first time they visit a cadaver lab. Years later, with vivid memories of my own initial visit intact, I returned to a gross anatomy laboratory. I had medical student housemates in graduate school and invited myself to their lab one day. I had learned about all sorts of muscles in my Rolfing pre-training. I figured if I could just get a close look at some of the little muscles around the spinal column, maybe I could figure out exactly what was bothering my back in particular, so I could fix it. No luck. They heaved a couple of heavily dissected cadavers into a sitting position (they were working on the belly) so I could view their backs. It was pretty bizarre. A very lively roomful of jovial young medical students busily taking very dead, embalmed human bodies apart. What was bizarre was how normal it seemed. Staring at dissected back muscles, I didn't gain any major insights on my own problem. What I did learn is that I am perfectly willing to endure some very strange versions of "normal" in my quest for knowledge.

By the time I was writing the dissertation, I had become good friends with another first-year medical student, and he invited me into the lab regularly on Saturdays when he went in to study for tests. I had a fairly good grasp of anatomy basics at this point. He and his teammates might have dissected an arm that week, and I would go in to see what they had accomplished. Since they were only doing one side, I would dissect the undone side myself while my friend prepared for his exam. This was quite an honor and I took it very seriously. I can still remember those initial cuts, knife parting flesh, on purpose. I had a real sense of the magnitude of my actions. I would go home from those sessions and endure the most awful dreams, oozing this and that. But the attraction somehow far outweighed my revulsion and I would find myself excitedly awaiting another opportunity to return to the lab and explore. I will remain forever grateful both to that friend who shared his cadaver with me, and to the woman who was so generous to have donated her body so that others could learn from it.

So that's how my journey into the body proceeded. I went back and forth between practical hands-on work with the living form, giving and receiving bodywork and practicing Tai Chi, to esoteric and spiritual readings and practices, to studying conventional science and medical textbooks. I could see from what I exposed myself to that there were certainly a wide variety of "takes" regarding the nature of the human form and its functions. I soaked them all in. I wasn't picky at that point. It was all recreation alongside my full-time research on the papal marriage teachings.

CHAPTER FOUR

Moving in Totally New Ways

That having been completed, I headed out to Colorado for the first of the two-phase Rolfing training. Now I could recreate full time. This was the summer of 1993, and I was twenty-nine years old. I had all but collected my diploma for the Ph.D., and I was embarking on a new career. I had not decided where I would live after the training. My student loans would not come due till the far side of graduation. I felt that kind of freedom you feel when you basically don't have any responsibilities except for yourself.

Little did I suspect I would meet the wife of my life on the first day of the training. She remembers her first impression of me: that I was some sort of posture-snob. I sat so rigidly in the class meeting circle, she figured I was trying to show off how upright my glorious, Rolfed body was. What she later learned was that I basically still endured constant, gnawing pain, despite all of my practices and inquiries. At least I wasn't stuck on the floor. I can't say I recall first impressions at all. I was coming out of a rather monkish period, having spent the bulk of the last year alone in a studio apartment reading and writing, coming out once a day to sweep the Coffee Shop and kibbitz with my friend, the building maintenance man. Now I was spending the whole day with twenty other people in class. They were an incredibly social bunch, that class. It took me a while to come out of my shell, but before long my front porch where I rented a room was a regular off-hours hang-out.

I hiked often in the rugged foothills of the Rockies. I tried weakly to keep up with my Tai Chi practices, but somehow they just didn't fit. This was odd to me, as I had been diligently practicing a couple of hours a day for the past five years. I was a "Tai Chi guy." The flowing forms of movement which I had learned and practiced for years had long given me a sense of inner calm. I had come to depend on them to rescue myself from bouts of back troubles, and focus my mind during years of intense study. Now, as I went through the movements, my mind would wander back to Chicago, where I had learned and practiced them. But I had intentionally moved on from there. Maybe I needed to let go of the Tai Chi practice as well. My head resisted. I valued the practice and had committed a lot of time and energy to learning what I knew, literally hours worth of movement sequences. Tai Chi felt like part of my identity. How could I just stop? The fact was, the practice had become a burden, and my body knew it. I didn't feel freed-up by the movements anymore. I just wanted to scramble around on the rocks in the mountains. It was as if the sequences which had originally expanded my repertoire of movement had become a rut and a limit-cycle in themselves. I wanted to move in different ways now. I slowly stopped practicing altogether, and never returned to it.

As for the training, it consisted of sitting and watching, sitting and watching. I went through the "old style" of Rolfing training, since changed dramatically for the better at the Rolf Institute. In the early seventies, Ida Rolf was teaching her students the work she had developed over many years. When one student just wasn't "getting it," she ordered him to sit and watch herself and others until he did. Thus was born the first phase of the training format. Teachers would work on clients while everyone watched, and advanced students would work on each other while beginners sat and watched. Finally, the advanced students would work on clients, while the beginners . . . sat and watched. This went on for over two months. It seemed that after a while, the only students who could stand to watch at all were the most cerebral, myself included. One by one, the beginners (aka "auditors") would leave for the bathroom or a smoke and stay out for as long as possible. Hand rolling cigarettes reached a fine art that summer. Eventually even non-smokers started puffing away outside, desperate for some distraction. There was simply too much watching to endure. I of course watched to the bitter end, so accustomed was I to sitting on my butt, ignoring my body, and staring at books and half-blank computer screens.

My apparent "availability" as an educated, single male with an undetermined future did not go unnoticed by some of the equally (or potentially) available women in the class. Such is the nature of many hours and weeks together in close quarters studying each other's bodies. In reaction, I made my "unavailability" as clear as possible. I even left my sexual orientation in question, if only to skew the availability issue even further. As far as I could see from a surface reading of myself, I was ready for a vacation from intimate relationships. The last one had been painful and the breakup difficult. I wanted to avoid enduring that sort of thing again soon. But I also held close to my heart an exchange I had some months back in Chicago with my therapist. I had said regarding the situation with my girlfriend that I could look only to myself for the difficult situation I was in with her. I said that I had clearly "vibrated" myself into the relationship. What would stop me from creating and repeating the same in the future? He responded that perhaps the reason I was so uncomfortable in the relationship was because I *was no longer* "vibrating" to it. We were growing apart. This was not a matter of one person being right or wrong, fair or unfair. It was simply the descriptive fact of the case. Perhaps that's why trying to stay together had become so painful for us, both emotionally and physically.

As the summer wore on I found myself sitting and watching one of my women classmates rather than the training sessions. Perhaps that's what kept me in the room for so long. She was beautiful, with long, mahogany-brown hair. She wore very funky clothing, baggy and cozy. If I could look into her past, I imagined a powerful, rooted Anasazi woman, an "old one" from the redlands of the southwest. Karen was an independent choreographer who funded her Philadelphia artist's life doing massage therapy, and was taking the next step in that career by becoming certified as a Rolfer. She was friendly and good-humored, and she had a man-friend back east. Oddly, I was becoming less interested in being alone most of the time in off-class hours, and began enjoying the social company of the class, Karen included. We became friends.

One night I had a dream. Karen and I, and several of our classmates were over at the Rolf Institute, joking and playing games and having a wonderful time. We had actually been doing as much on a regular basis. I guess I had to dream it to wake up to how much fun I was having. I awoke incredibly refreshed, renewed in the experience of how easy it could be to be in relationship with someone. I could have fun with Karen! One weekend her man-friend came to town. I knew they were on somewhat rocky ground, and must admit I was not rooting for their eternal bliss together. I was out with the gang, and we crossed paths with them on a side-walk on Friday night and were all introduced. In that moment my hopes abounded. One look and I could tell they were in a similar situation to what I had recently left. They were moving on differ-ent paths, and not "co-vibrating." The next night we all went out to see the film, "Like Water for Chocolate." Her man-friend was off with other acquaintances. With rich cinematography and storytelling, the tale explores themes of supportive friendship and passionate love. For the main characters, the two experiences seem excluded to different relationships. Leaving the theater, Karen asked me if I thought it was possible to find both with the same person. "Sure!" I said, and I believed it, looking at her.

Not long after, Karen returned from a visit to her man-friend a "single" woman again. They had gone to a wedding and it had become obvious to her that it was time to move on. We spent more time together as friends. I had made it so clear that I was not interested in a relationship to other women in the class, Karen assumed from the rumor mill that I meant what I said. I had never mentioned that I would gladly renege on my "commitment" to the single life for her, given how I had come to feel for her. But I still had my own reservations. What held me back? I had wrestled with so many issues surrounding my own family life. As surely as I didn't want an immediate repeat performance of my last relationship, I didn't want to repeat my first seventeen years anytime soon, either. I was suffering from "fear of family" syndrome. I visited my parents and sisters periodically. But I had kept my family at an emotional and physical distance for quite some time. My sisters had four children apiece. I enjoyed being an uncle, but for all of my willingness to *think* about marriage, I could never imagine myself as a parent. And now my parents were planning a visit to see me in Colorado. I had received their plans rather tepidly. From a distance, I had always told my parents that I loved them. Living it out in close-quarters had not been in my immediate plans.

I shared my concerns with my classmate/housemate/buddy. He had mentioned his folks were planning a visit as well. I thought we would commiserate. Beware where you look for someone to collude with you in your fears and anxieties. He slammed me so hard with a half-hour long diatribe it made my head spin. St. Thomas taught that a strong medicine can put you on the road to health. This speech was just what the doctor ordered. He upbraided me thoroughly, telling me what a whining brat I sounded like. "So, your childhood wasn't perfect! So, your parents weren't exactly how you think they should have been! Well, they didn't kill you! You don't look so much the worse for it all, Mr. Duke graduate, Mr. Ph.D. What do you want from them? Wasn't four years of wiping your butt enough? And they love you and want to see you, you little snot. Get over it! Call them up, and beg them to come here. Tell them you love them and can't wait to see them, and when they get here, show them the town and have a great time. They did their best with what they knew, and it's about time you quit your sniveling infantile resentments and grew up!"

Any protests of my own against his words suddenly sounded ridiculous and empty. I had been playing the child-victim and it was a very unsatisfying role. Venting about my parents was no more fulfilling than venting about the popes. In fact, it was the exact same thing. I had begun to grow up in my faith, somehow. Now I could become an adult relative to my parents as well. I felt ashamed at the way I had held my parents at arms-length over my petty resentments for so long. But shame was not my motivating factor for literally running down the stairs to use the phone immediately after my friend had given me the full dose. I was excited to make new choices about how I would be with my parents, and to follow them up with action.

It turned out they never did make the trip, and I was honestly disappointed. Nonetheless, my consciousness had been raised a couple of notches, with positive repercussions. I felt free to love. Holding back my love for my parents was nothing more than that: me holding back *my experience of love.* Blaming someone else for my problems was a choice, regardless of what anyone else "had done." Playing the role of the victim was a choice that deprived me of my own experience of loving fully. I was tired of whining.

Turning towards Karen with this understanding, I knew I had nothing to fear. I would allow myself to love her, and if it worked out for the long run, great. If it didn't, well, it certainly did feel good to love her freely in the short run. I no longer saw any value in holding back. "Honor your father and your mother" had never made more sense. At this point we were to the last week of the training. My housemate invited Karen and me to stroll into the nearby mountains to watch the meteor showers late one evening. The night was moonless with incredibly bright stars, which seemed periodically to dislodge from their orbits and streak across the sky with flashes of light.

My roomate somehow convinced us (was this a setup?) that the whole experience would definitely be even more fun if we took in the meteor shower "in the buff," so we laid our cloths out on the ground for "blankets" and gazed up at nature's display while displaying our own nature back to it. After taking in the sights for a long time, we dressed to go. Expansion, contraction. It seems I had laid out my bed of clothing on a bed of cactus, and as I put them back on I was skewered with innumerable tiny super-fine needles. I spent the rest of the night and the next day in class un-pin-cushioning *every* part of my anatomy. Youch.

After a bonding experience like that, I was wanting to make it more clear to Karen how I felt about her, given the doubts I had sown about my openness to an intimate relationship. So I asked her to make a batch of "Gil's" cookie dough with me in preparation for the party that would celebrate the close of our training. Remember, I am the guy who once gave a laundry basket to his girlfriend for her birthday. We went to the store one evening, picked up the ingredients, rented *Conan the Barbarian* at the video store (I still loved Arnold, despite long having given up weight training), and went back to her place to mix dough. It was late when we finally got to the movie, and with endless commentaries, we laughed out loud through the whole thing. Now it was 2am. I had hopes for a generous offer to sack out with the great company, but instead she offered me a lift home. That *was* a generous offer, given I otherwise would have had to walk about six miles in the middle of the night. Beyond making cookie dough and watching *Conan*, how much more obvious could I possibly make my affection for her?

The next night we had plans to get more friends together to watch the ongoing meteor shower. Somehow everyone else bagged out, and we were left to our own devices. This time we brought a thick blanket to guard against the cacti, and kept our clothes on. The night was cool, and with no one else around, we were a bit giddy and shy. We snuggled on the blanket and watched stars shoot between the clouds. Our hands found each other's. It remains to this day a lively source of debate between us exactly who "doodled" the other's fingers first. As our hands met while we watched the stars, I for my part perceived a distinct doodling of my fingers on her part, which led me to believe she indeed had a romantic interest in me. Would you doodle someone's fingers who was "just" a friend? Nah. She insists *I* doodled *her* fingers and that's how she knew *I* was interested in a romantic relationship. But I *never* would have doodled first. Although neither of us will admit to having doodled first (she did!), we both agree that believing the other to have done so set us officially on our path to union. Looking at her there in the foothills of the Rockies it occurred to me I could imagine this woman being the mother of my children. I can barely convey how novel that thought was for me. I married Karen in my heart that night, and although we didn't "tie the knot" in public for another ten months, we have been marrying each other on a daily basis ever since.

The first half of our Rolfing training was ended and our relationship had only just begun. I decided to stay in New Jersey at my folks' house, until the second part. Karen was returning to Philly before her second training in Florida. Hers was in five weeks, mine in five months, in California. Since we had only been "a couple" for literally one day, despite our giddiness I hardly knew how to imagine things working out between us as a practical matter. I flew back to New Jersey excitedly telling my family about my new friend. I was feeling wonderful. Karen was driving for three days straight back to the East Coast for a dance performance at the Lincoln Center, and had promised to call. When I was told the phone was for me, I went to it like a puppy for chow. But no one was on the line. All I could hear was some crackling and some music, and then the caller hung up. I figured the coffee clutch gang from class was just teasing me, and it happened just that way several more times. I was a mess. Here my friends were torturing me, and I hadn't heard from Karen. I figured I had just set a new personal record for speedily flubbed relationships.

Karen finally called when she got in to Philly. I was thrilled to hear from her. I reported my strange ordeal. Knowing she would never have done as much, I told her our friends were messing with my mind, and asked what kept her from calling earlier. She got giggly. As it turns out, she had been listening to love songs for two thousand miles, periodically pulling off the road to play them for me as a romantic treat, serenading me with the lyrics. Blasting her car radio into pay phones on the side of the highway took its toll on sound quality, and my beloved's messages had gone unheard.

Well, that was a relief. I watched her performance in New York City a couple of days later with wonderment, and brought her home to meet the family. Little did she realize her visit fell on some occasion for a party. Eight nieces and nephews, two recently born whom I was meeting myself for the first time, family friends, my sisters, their husbands, my parents. No pressure! Just be yourself! Karen was holding babies, doing dishes, the works. Realize this was basically our third date. My sisters whisked up to me to offer their candid (exuberant) evaluations. One offered her wedding dress as a loaner. At least I wasn't the only one prone to jumping to conclusions.

We were inseparable. Either I drove down to Philly or she came back to New Jersey. Given my interest in Barbara Brennen's work, I had enrolled in her school's introductory workshop in Washington, D.C., and we stayed with Karen's parents this time. Now it was my turn. They were no more prone to hiding their judgments than my family: I was plainly an answer to their prayers for Karen, as far as they could see. No pressure there either! I knew the old saying, if you want to know what your wife will look like in thirty years, look at her mother. Her mother was adorable, and a good hugger too. I figured I was set.

I spoke a lot with Karen about my interest in the work of energy healers. She came to the open lecture of the weekend workshop with Barbara Brennen. Then she joined me for a weekend in New York City which was meant to introduce another school for energetic healing based there. I wanted to compare the two, and perhaps attend the school that attracted me the most after I completed the Rolfing training. I wanted to explore my spirituality as well as psychic phenomena, my body, and my growing touch-skills. This kind of exploration was new to Karen, but she moved into it so easily I could barely keep up. Karen had left spirituality behind with the Catholic Church in which she was raised. She saw me still attending mass regularly, and exploring spiritual questions constantly. We started going to Church together and spoke often about matters of life and spirit, scripture and Church. The healing schools seemed another step in that direction which we could take together.

We surprised ourselves with the power of our experiences at the introductory workshop for the IM School of Healing Arts, based in SOHO at the time. The school's founder had worked for five years with Brennan and eventually started his own program, giving him the freedom to develop his own teaching style. I enjoyed the program but didn't feel ready to make the financial commitment. Karen was more deeply smitten, and determined to come back somehow. By this time I had arranged to go to Florida with Karen and participate in the training there with her. That would place us together for the next three months at least. After that, who could say? We set up to live with two other friends-in-training in a rental condo on the Gulf of Mexico and commute to the Tampa class. Days before the long drive South, we were frolicking in a public pool. I was showing off for my new love, feeling like a teenager, and doing flips from the diving board. On my final launch, I flopped instead of flipped. I crawled out of the water with the familiar dreadful knifelike pain in my upper back. I could feel my body contracting from that place with nasty severity. By the time we got home I was twisted around myself like a human corkscrew. I sobbed like a baby as Karen iced the area. I was in physical pain, but also emotionally thunderstruck. How could I have worked so hard at understanding my body and improving myself, and still have the same problem? I dreaded the prospect of spending the rest of my life moving cautiously, in fear of further injury.

By the time we got to Florida I was still looking bent out of shape and moving with caution, but the immediate severity had been traded for dull pain. Here I had come, once again, to learn how to help people feel and move with greater bodily ease, and I was actually afraid to get more work myself. I worried that my training partner would do me under as a novice in the art of Rolfing. My experience was quite the opposite of my fears. With the guidance of our teacher, my training partner gently led me over the weeks to a much better place, and six years later I've never endured anything quite like those miserable episodes again.

During this part of the training, after a couple of weeks of anatomy review and movement studies, we Rolfed each other as well as clients. No more watching for weeks on end. Three days into the second week, Karen and another friend were late returning from lunch. After ten minutes, I was nervous. After fifteen, I was panicked. My mother was the type who called the police and local hospitals if we were half an hour late. To add to our concern, my partner had heard sirens a few minutes earlier. We sent a class assistant out on the road to look for them. She returned having found the totaled wreckage of Karen's car and the bloodied scene of an accident being cleared from the road. Karen and our housemate had been rushed in ICU ambulances to the emergency room at Tampa General.

The whole class piled into cars and rushed to the hospital. After what seemed like an eternity, I was ushered in as "next of kin" to where they were being treated. Karen was coming out of shock, with various trickling cuts and bruises. She was strapped to a board with her head braced, shards of glass matted into her bloodied hair. She was very glad to see me but her only concern was our other friend, and the driver of the other car (he was able to walk from the scene on his own). Karen had been driving and was broadsided crossing an intersection by someone who technically had the right-of-way. She never saw him coming. That's why they call them accidents. They had gone out to shop for a present for me for my birthday the next day. I checked on our injured friend in the next room. She was in that punchy stage of a concussion, repeating the same questions over and over again, trying to figure out where she was, how she got there, the names of her pets and husband, and what country we were in (she was born in Germany but married an American). She was also strapped up and required stitches in various places. Her only real concern was for Karen. Neither of them could remember my assurances that the other was OK for more than a moment, so I went back and forth between the two rooms, answering to the one's delirium and assuring them the other was all right.

I for my part was a wreck. It was apparent that the trauma was disorienting for the two of them, but I later realized how disorienting the field of trauma was for me as well. The emergency room treatment area was set up completely for the "practicalities" of stapling someone back together, but the aesthetic needs of those same "someones" went completely unanswered. As Karen was wheeled out for CAT scans and x-rays, I sat alone in the gray-walled room under cool-white fluorescent lights, feeling utterly desolate. The various medical appliances and accoutrements had nothing to say. I headed back to play twenty questions with our friend while interns stitched her lacerated ear. Meanwhile, the interns quizzed me on Rolfing. They seemed happy that someone could answer this woman's endless stream of confused questions. This was all in a day's work, and they were quite innocently passing the time with me. Eventually, they wheeled her off to the intensive care unit to monitor her concussion, and I returned to Karen's side an expert in confirming the name of Champ the dog, Chris the husband, and the State of Florida. I will never forget the conversation, and developed a deep compassion for the mentally confused on the spot.

Karen was brought to a room for the night, where I stayed until the nurse kicked me out some time after visiting hours had ended. It was late when she got there. The nurse announced (without irony) that Karen was in luck, because the hospital kitchen was closed, and she was free to order whatever she wanted from the McDonald's restaurant downstairs. This to a woman who lived on fresh organic foods and gourmet coffees. She went for the McFish and tossed the bun. Karen is of the belief that the American penchant for fluffy white buns is rooted in the low levels of breast-feeding in our country. If we were breast-fed more as babies, she reasons, we would be less inclined to be constantly nuzzling those soft fluffy buns (while sucking sweet sodas from straws, I might add).

If we had been in need of bonding, this pretty much covered it. Convinced that the two of them would survive the night, I caught a ride with some kind soul, a friend of the inquiring class assistant who lived nearby (we housemates were commuting an hour to the coast twice daily). I awoke the next morning (my thirtieth birthday) and headed straight back to the hospital. Karen was being released, while our friend remained in intensive care. We had all prayed incessantly for their healing since the moment we knew of the accident. I called on Jesus and Mary and the angels and saints, wise teachers who had passed on, and anyone else who wanted to help a couple of women in need. My pantheon of spiritual guides remains heavily populated still. They were clearly busy at our behest. Our friend was sitting up in ICU, laughing about her questions of the day before, and thankful Karen was on her feet. Actually my smart mouth was now trouble, as their broken and bruised ribs pained them from any laughter.

Karen was on her feet, however wobbly. But on our way back to the condo, it became clear that all was not well. By the time we'd gotten home, Karen was covered with red welts, hives, and she was itching like Job. We found a clinic and the doctor prescribed lindane, an incredibly toxic pesticide used to treat scabies, an itchy pest. We doused ourselves and the bedding to no avail. This itch was no bug, and wouldn't budge. Karen actually itched continuously for the following three years. That's a long time to be scratching. The Itch, we called it. Our friend joined us the next day, to our relief. The two were healing in body virtually before our eyes, despite the fact that they were having some difficulty staying in them. They actually remained disoriented for months, to some extent. Remember that the next time you meet someone coming out of an accident. They are rarely all there. Memory lapses and returns, fog comes and goes.

Our friend reported that two nights in a row she had had extremely vivid dreams of people coming to teach her certain principles and techniques of self healing from the accident, as well as suggestions for protecting herself in the future. I had actually been calling on a particular Greek Cypriot healer and his accomplices to help us. We marveled at the correlation of style between the dreams and the folks I was "tuning" to. Help that practical was more than I had anticipated, and we felt supported in ways not normally recognized.

We all resumed the training despite the persistent effects of the accident. Karen was possessed by the itch and we spent most of our off hours and days desperately trying to effect a cure. We went to accupuncturists, experimented with diet, applied topical prescriptions, and generally obsessed about it. Then I drank Karen's contact lenses. The glass of water on the night table had looked awfully innocent to me. Her glasses had been broken in the accident, and we hadn't replaced them yet. Now she was basically blind, bruised and scratching. For some reason it took nearly a week to replace her eyeglass prescription. She turned way inside in desperation. And folks in class wondered why she seemed a little difficult to connect with at the time. This was the bad day that wouldn't quit. We like to say that as far as "for better or for worse" goes, we started with for worse, and it's been getting better ever since.

CHAPTER FIVE

Giving Up the Fight

For my part, I was in puppy love and glad to be with Karen. Even at her self-perceived worst, she was easy to live with. Our other two condo-mates were also great friends. Despite our trials, we enjoyed watching dolphins and great blue herons from our balcony. We took long walks together on the beach when we weren't in class or dealing with the itch. My pelvis was also awakening from its long slumber. Between the additional Rolfing work and the good company, more movement was percolating within my stifled body. I was also reading, of course. At this point I was deeply enamored by a series of three books written by Kyriacos Markides about the esoteric Christian healer from Cyprus known as Daskolos, whom I mentioned in passing above.

I actually read the three books three times apiece! Here was a fellow who referred to the human brain as "that clump of earth inside your skull." Pretty cocky, I thought. Daskolos' worldview was that of someone who had waked up from the dream of daily life. People in general, myself included most of the time, tend to operate with the belief that what you see of this physical world is pretty much what there is to deal with. Daskolos, not unlike Barbara Brennan or Castaneda's teacher, claimed to see many more layers of the world, and considered the physical world as just one of many "planes" on which we operate, whether we are conscious of it or not. And if we do become conscious of it, it is best the awareness grow with a sense of responsibility, as there is as much service to be done as mistakes to be made. I was reminded of my "out-of-body" attempt. Daskolos claimed to have the ability to do this at will, but his intent was centered on service and teaching, versus my vague curiosity at the time.

Reading those books, I felt the desire burning even more deeply to let the way I typically experienced things crumble. This multi-layered worldview made sense to me intuitively, despite the limits of my personal experience. Sure, I had this physical body. But how the heck did it even move around? I had learned much of the very basic mainstream scientific information available on muscle physiology. The brain and spinal cord stimulate muscles, and there are feedback loops back to the central nervous system from the muscles. The complexity of the pathways back and forth was truly breathtaking. I admired the persistence of the people who spent years in laboratories trying to figure out the inside story which I now took for granted. Still, as told by mainstream science, the story is a relatively short one. It has virtually nothing to say about the will, or the motivations of movement. The mind is usually reduced to electrical discharges in the physical brain, which can be vaguely mapped and measured with scans and EEGs.

For Daskolos, the Divine Mind and our developing consciousness were the key players. The brain and physical processes in general were more like mere "hard copies" of the choices and activities and levels of awareness of the maturing human being. He did not place the brain in charge. After all, even the "voluntary" bodily movements which mainstream science describes imply a "will" directing the physical brain. So what does physical science have to say about the "will?" Pretty much nothing. For that you need to turn to the social sciences, or religion, or ethics—mushy science—not really science at all, according to some. "Involuntary" movements, like the beating of one's heart or the processes of digestion, are things that, on a good day, happen *automatically* according to biological science. They are out of "conscious" control, according to the same mainstream science that generally refuses to address or even ask what consciousness is in the first place.

Reading Daskolos, my ideas about bodily movement learned

from scientific studies got turned upside down. For one thing, he and many others out there seemed to have become quite conscious of those unconscious processes and learned to direct them at will. Marvelous accounts of yoga practitioners heating up their naked bodies under wet blankets in the snow point to the simpler truth about the role of our will in so called "involuntary" physical processes. I can remember visiting my dad in an intensive care unit once when he was hospitalized. He had me watch the monitor and proudly demonstrated his ability to change his blood-oxygen levels at will, just by focusing on his breathing. This is the basis of "biofeedback" therapies, which some have raised to a very fine art.

Furthermore, those so-called "voluntary" movements are only "in my control" in the broadest sense. At more basic physical levels, willfulness and choice seem remote. You can call squeezing your thumb on the clicker to change the channel "voluntary" if you want. But thank God you don't have to know all of the complex chemistry, physics, biology, and kinesiology which underlie that simple act before you could perform it, or you'd be watching the same station for the rest of your life. Daskolos was keen to point out that we are not acting alone in our bodies. For him, the tremendous complex intricacies and processes of life in physical form were the domain of nature spirits, devas and archangelic entities who were the masters of the elements. The incredible intelligence of the human body reflected the mastery of these co-operating intelligences, who themselves acted in accord with the "Divine Will-Pleasure."

At our service and the service of all creation and the Divine Mind, these intelligences took care of matters beyond the grasp and limits of our intellect and normal mental processes. In doing so, they leave us free to develop and mature in those matters over which we are duly appointed, namely the growth and maturing of our own "petty time-and-place personalities," our emotions and our spiritual selves. By inspecting and working to resolve our own underdeveloped or problematic areas, and capitalizing on our strengths, we can move towards an experience of body, emotions, mind and spirit integrated together in a unified manner, in coop-eration with those supporting intelligences. That's when the work really begins. For Daskolos, it wasn't simply a matter of "getting it together" for your own sake exclusively. The fruit of the work of introspection and personal integration is just the starting point of service to one's fellows, all creation, and the Divine Life. Develop-ing one's own integrity results in the desire and responsibility to serve the integration of the larger whole.

Part of what I liked about becoming a Rolfer was that I felt if I was to grow as a practitioner, I would have to grow as a person as well. If I was to lead people to a more integrated experience of their body and their life, I had to lead by example as well as by touch. By claiming to practice "structural integration," the ge-neric term for what Rolfer's do, I was putting myself on the spot to "walk the talk," and I wanted that for myself. However, Karen and I both noticed that the limited time-frame of our training, with so much on the agenda in terms of the principles and practical tech-niques of Rolfing, didn't leave much room for exploring introspec-tion and personal development at these other important levels. We were ready to collect our "title," but still we wanted to learn more about the integration of the whole person, for ourselves in the first place.

Our thoughts turned to the healing school back in SOHO, 1300 miles to the north. The group from our introductory class would be meeting for a weekend the very next day after the comple-tion of our Rolfing training. We hadn't replaced Karen's car, we didn't know how we would pay for the school, and a reasonably priced flight on such short notice seemed out of the question. But strange things were pointing us there anyway. One of our class-mates had an odd experience on more than one occasion, hearing a distant voice calling repeatedly for Karen. We made what we wanted of that: a Sign! Then I got a phone call from a friend, saying she had a dream that Karen and I had really enjoyed our intro week-end at the healing school, and that it seemed likely we would go, and not to worry about financing it. I learned of a local airline that had no-advanced-purchase flights for only $89 from Tampa to Newark, New Jersey.

We concluded from these signs and wonders that it was our mutual destiny to attend the healing school, packed our bags, and were literally driven by our friends straight from graduation to the airport. Unfortunately, when we got to the gate, our reservation was nowhere to be found in the computer. We only had a moment to be crestfallen, however. The ticketing agent (who also worked the flight, and who may have been the pilot and sole owner for all we knew) informed us that we could board the plane immediately for $69 apiece. So much for advanced planning. We took the forty dollar savings as a divine confirmation, and boarded the plane. It may be a wicked age that seeks a sign, but we'll take what we can get anyway.

Throughout our time in Florida, Karen and I had further grown on and with each other, and were inseparable. At the very least, we had committed to establishing a Rolfing practice together in New Jersey or Philadelphia. Now we were taking on the healing school. We were including ourselves in each other's futures, but hadn't dared to pronounce the "M" word to each other. We had only been together as a couple for three and a half months, after all. Our friends from the healing school still kid us that when we all met at the introductory weekend, they had assumed Karen and I had been "together" for several years. In fact, it had only been three weeks at the time since we had thrown our lots in with each other. We still marvel that we found each other. We must have planned that back in heaven.

We loved the weekend in Manhattan, commuting from my folks' house in New Jersey in a borrowed car. The school was very casual. With a group of thirty people or so sitting in a circle and flopped about on pillows and couches, we began what grew into a continually deeper exploration of ourselves, the way we choose to present ourselves to the world, and the heart of our inner nature. We were now a pair of homeless Rolfers, smitten with each other, embarking on what turned out to be a four year long healer's training. Although we committed to the program year by year, from that early time we had a sense that we would be in it for the long haul.

For the first two years we met for seven three-day weekends each year. The second two years we were there even more often, assisting the earlier classes as well as attending our own. All in all I figure we spent nearly 40 weekends at the school. That's a lot of time sitting in a circle, and I don't regret a single day of it. The real irony is that I was never one for circles. As far back as my pre-training at the Rolf Institute, I can remember that the only thing I ever said in that kind of group discussion was "I hate circles!" But a couple of things made the circles at the healing school different. I grew in my trust of my friends and teachers, and I slowly stopped feeling the need to be perceived as "right."

What, after all, drives a person to plow through seven years of graduate studies in ethics, if not a compulsion to be right about something? While I will never regret my years in graduate school, reflecting back upon them I recognize how deeply important it was for me to be "right" about the teachings with which I was wrestling. And even if the pope didn't agree with me, I had to be right in my own head at the very least. Needing to be right or perceived as right can seem to be virtually a matter of life or death for the person struggling with it. I felt a real sense of desperation around it. Wrong is bad, right is good, bad is shameful, good rewarding. These polarities drove me, and sitting in those circles I slowly came to understand how.

I can remember the anxiety that would rise up in me when someone said something that was apparently "wrong to me." My mind would race. I felt compelled from within to correct the wrong, hearing nothing in the conversation until I had uttered my version of the truth. And if I felt someone had misperceived my version of the truth, I would feel equally compelled to clarify what I had said over and over in the hopes of convincing anyone and everyone (who could still stand to listen) regarding exactly what I had meant. I found it incredibly exhausting to "have to" try to control the perceptions of everyone in the circle, but was at a loss for quite some time not to. I really felt the need for everyone to think I was right/good. Remembering my great awakening in college when I perceived and experienced my essential goodness, you would think I'd have developed a different take on this, but certain basic issues of character run very deep, and demand serious attention more than once over the course of a lifetime.

This was directly related to winning and losing, and my dad and I shared this trait like genes. Winning is good, losing is bad. This is just one step towards *winners* are good, and losers are bad, winners are right, losers are wrong. My dad is an expert game player. Tell him the basic rules, and he'll figure them out and dominate you perpetually after the first few rounds. As a child, I always loved playing games (and losing them) with my dad, but after a while I stopped playing all together. I told myself I hated competition. I joined the high school track team three years in a row only to quit when the competitive part of the season began. I wasn't in it to win or lose, I told myself.

I was attracted to weightlifting, where I could compete against gravity, the mirror, and the tape measure, but never anyone else. I loved bicycling, competing with my wristwatch and the road. With Tai Chi, again, it was my own wits that I challenged as I perfected the movements. The drive to compete was in me, but I kept it directed towards my own development. By avoiding competition with others, I sidestepped the problem of winning or losing altogether. Or so I thought. In college, a professor, probably the most intimidating one I had ever had, told me privately one day that *I* was intimidating the other students in our seminar. He would have known. I realized that when I was engaging in some kind of argument with another student in class, I went for the jugular, and fought to win with the same inner ferocity I had seen in my dad. My personal style was to kill them more or less kindly, without them knowing I was in the process of pulling the rug out from under them and their ideas. I had been voted the friendliest guy in my high school class, after all. I didn't realize the life or death stakes I had placed on winning, and being right, or at least perceived as right, until a couple of years into the healing school, nearly half a lifetime later.

If I had to be right to be good, and good to deserve to live, then you can be damn sure I would fight to be right. The flip side of this was that if I was actually wrong about something, or someone perceived me as wrong about something, boy, did I feel bad. That would shake me to the core. I had never suspected all of this at the roots of my quest for sanctity. But my quest for holiness was as much about the neurotic anxiety I felt about being right or wrong as it was a sincere aspiration for God in my life. You can tell when the need to be right is neurotic when, even after you win the argument or other people agree with you, the victory feels sort of hollow. The position of needing to be right/good/to win was incredibly insecure. It depended on other people's perceptions, some of whom may have needed to be right as much as I did.

Once I got into an argument with my dad when I was back from college. I was actually on my way to church on a Sunday morning. Before getting out the door, we were baiting and switching about the Reagan presidency and associated matters like two jackals come upon a kill. There was no way I was backing down, however ridiculous my statements were becoming. We went back and forth snapping at each other until to my utter surprise dad, red as a beet, shouted "You win!" and stomped out of the room. I felt horrible. I honestly worried that I'd nearly killed the man on the spot, verbally. It was the first (and last) time I had ever fought in one of those battles with him to "victory." I had lots to think about at Church *that* morning. A huge gap had opened up before me between winning and being "right," on the one side, and being good on the other. I sure as heck didn't feel good winning that one. I didn't figure it out on the spot, but I never allowed myself to reach quite that fever pitch with my dad again. I did at least become suspicious that proving oneself "right" might give rise to "winning," but not necessarily goodness. The equation of the three was off.

Sometime during the second year in the healing school, I started to hear the tinny sound of some of the things I said. I began to notice when I got anxious to "correct" someone or something. I started to realize that I was incredibly uncomfortable and felt miserable in my body whenever I thought someone mistook something I said, or even something someone else said to another, totally unrelated to me. I became deeply suspicious of my urgent need to make everything right, because the compulsion to do so felt so bad. Speaking from anxiety and urgency also lacks the same impact as something offered solidly from the heart. Recognition was and is a big step towards healing. It's pretty tough to make a new choice about something if you don't recognize the unconscious choices you've been making in the first place.

I am still working with the issue, but I have achieved some milestones. You may as well know that at this point I have come to consider myself a self-styled entrepreneur, happily married. Now there's a shift for someone who spent most of his life expecting to make vows of poverty, chastity and obedience. Who says people can't change? My main entrepreneurial endeavor is teaching continuing education workshops in anatomy for allied health professionals of all sorts. More on how that came about later. A couple of years ago, I taught two consecutive classes which shared a common event. In both classes, particular students made it perfectly and vehemently clear that they thought I was "wrong" about something. Now, for some of you reading this, that might not sound like a big deal. But given what I have described above, you may have an idea of the challenge this posed for me. My standard options historically had been either to collapse in shame because I was "bad," or to fight back with some sort of self-justifying retort, tit for tat. Somehow I had the fortitude in the moment to just sit and listen as best I could. In the second instance, other students stepped in to defend me, but by then I realized the importance of remaining undefended. I did not want accomplices either.

As a teacher, and as a person wanting healing, I knew how destructive it could be to even passively permit my defense and the subsequent division of the class. I actually did not want to defend myself as right or good, nor did I want anyone to do it for me. Now don't get me wrong, it's not like I didn't have second thoughts! But I had grown in the conviction that in order for *me* to feel good *in myself*, in my own body, I had to relinquish my compulsion to prove myself right to the world, and my need to control the perceptions of others in that direction. I made another choice. I have since had various successes and failures with this, but I also know that my essential goodness, rightness, and ultimate victory is independent of the hopeless struggles in which I have engaged. I am good, because God is good in me. When I am aligned with the Divine presence within myself, I quite honestly need no defense. I once read, and I believe, that the truth needs no defense. I am convinced that the truth lies beyond the argument, beyond the divisions of right and wrong, beyond winning and losing, winners and losers, and the scales of bad and "good." Now when I am afraid of losing an argument, that is my cue that I have stepped out of alignment with the truth.

Having returned to the Northeast, Karen and I decided that since we were going into a Rolfing practice together, we wanted to live together too. We had become both lovers and best friends, and couldn't imagine it otherwise. We were committed to setting "Like Water for Chocolate" straight: you really can have both friendship and passion in the same relationship. We used my folks' place as a launch point to search for the perfect office and the perfect housing situation. We scoured the towns and newspapers, looking for a place close enough to commute to the healing school, and pleasant enough to live. We were spoiled after a summer in Boulder and autumn on the beaches of the Gulf.

My parents were cordial, and Karen's presence and easy way with my folks created a balance to my relationship with them that I hadn't had the last time I had lived with them. A lot had changed in me, and I was ready and willing to reincorporate my family into my life more fully. But some of those changes were a bit scary for my mother. When I was in my good and pious Catholic saint wannabee stage, she at least understood the basic rules. She could see how my extremism was distorted, but the basic picture looked right. Now the basic picture was looking distorted from her vantage as well. I was talking about lucid dreaming, out of body travel, reincarnation, healing energy, channeling, and the like. It all sounded a bit scary and devilish to her. This from the woman who had once woken in the middle of the night to see the wall of the tent in which she was sleeping dissolve before her eyes to behold a throng of "angels" passing by.

Frankly, if you've ever read some of the stuff that Catholic saints have been into, I hadn't strayed too far from the path. Some of those folks were pretty wacky. But my language was scaring her. It's one thing to believe in "angels," but "spirit guides" are out of the question. And reincarnation? That was clearly against the Church's teachings. Don't mind the fact that it was commonly believed for the first three hundred years of Christianity at least, and was taught by the beloved fathers of the Church. And what was it Jesus said about Elijah "coming back?" He said he has come back, as John the Baptizer. I haven't heard a whole lot of sermons lately on that verse!

To be honest, I probably meant to scare her a bit, however unconscious I was of the behavior and intent. I was wanting to be closer to my parents, but I was still operating out of old resentments and fears. My new habits towards them were growing, but poorly formed. There was still an aggressive edge to the way I presented my new explorations to my mother which needed to be sanded down. After one of these conversations, she told me she didn't like where I was going with my life in all of this. I was hurt, and returned to the conversation an hour later to say that she didn't have the foggiest idea where my life was going, and that I was on a wonderful path of discovery upon which I hoped she'd join me. But, if she wanted to stay with her fear, I was going nonetheless. It was a turning point for me to take a stance so strong relative to hers, and marked a step in my growth as an independent person. The vastly bigger step, which I took much more gradually, was to understand and temper the hostilities that bubbled about inside of me. Eventually I came to the point where I could speak without attempting to intimidate her regarding the things about which I was so excited. All it really took was paying attention to how much I loved her, rather than rehashing in my mind what I wanted her to be or do.

CHAPTER SIX

The Incarnation Project

My folks generously invited us to stay with them and keep our overhead low while we built our Rolfing practice, and we took them up on it. We really did enjoy each other's company. My dad, retired, took up the responsibility of cooking nightly for the up-start Rolfers and his working wife. I hadn't eaten so well in years. I began feeling heartier. Nothing like getting some good red meat into a chronic bean-eater. Karen and I had been coached by one of our teachers regarding an office for our practice: "If you build it, they will come—so make your office really nice." Since we didn't have any clients to work on, and our housing situation was re-solved for the time being, we threw ourselves into finding a place out of which to build a practice. We picked a huge office in down-town Westwood, New Jersey, and ignored the heavy price, figur-ing our practice would build fast since we had such an awesome office. Such are the kinds of decisions made by people with no real business sense and lots of excitement. We spent hours and hours re-upholstering antique furniture, painting, framing pictures, and generally spending every last cent on our office. Then we would count how much money we were going to have with two of us having full practices. Unfortunately, this turned out to be the snowi-est winter on record for years. We scheduled talk after talk, plaster-ing the town with fliers for people to come learn about Rolfing. Then we would sit watching the snow falling outside our office, and after an hour or so we would put our brochures and things away and schedule the next "demo." Once one guy actually came.

You would have thought he was a bag of groceries, we were so excited at the prospect of having a client. He endured a heavy sell job, but never did come for a session.

Finally some advertising in a community paper paid off, and we started to get some business. At eighty bucks a session, we were feeling pretty good. But with rent at $1100 a month, and lots more invested, we soon realized we were in over our heads. Rolfing Associates closed its downtown doors three months after the grand opening, and we learned a huge lesson in keeping the overhead of a new business as low as possible. We still tease our teacher about his advice. Now he suggests starting a fledgling practice on a shoestring. Having faced the decision of closing the office or quitting the healing school, we knew which we preferred. And thanks once again to the bottomless support of my parents, we were invited to take over a front room in the house which suited our needs to a tee. We were also driving a car which replaced Karen's wreck, courtesy of her parents. Being the beneficiary of the largesse of both sets of parents kept us afloat at the time. Nonetheless, our debts were mounting faster than ever. We were using our earnings to pay for the healing school, while watching the numbers add up on the credit card. As we joined our lives, we joined our finances too. That is to say, we added her debts to my Ph.D. debts, Piled hi and Deep.

We had also gotten engaged on New Year's Eve, four months after I had committed in my own mind and heart to marry Karen. I figured I'd have to give her more than the one day it took me to decide. Of course I had been casting out the "M" word like bait on a hook for months, seeing if she would nibble. I wasn't about to bring it up for real unless I had a pretty decent inkling that she wanted to marry me as well, despite her comical unwillingness to say the word "marriage." We had gone to my sister's on New Year's Eve to baby sit four of my nieces and nephews while they went to a party. What more perfect a setting to pop the question? After the kids were asleep we snuggled before a cozy fire and I proposed to Karen that we marry each other on a daily basis for the rest of our lives. *That* was fun, despite the whole body flutter it took to get those words out of my mouth. Thank God she said yes. It would have been a real downer watching "the ball" drop at midnight if she hadn't. Happy New Year!

Both our families were delighted if not surprised. We set a date in June, two weeks after I was to be granted my Ph.D. in graduation ceremonies back in Chicago. Between starting our practice, closing our office, Rolfing our clients, making wedding plans, growing in our relationship, attending the healing school and graduating, we had a lot on our plate. I felt as if my life was starting to hit stride. I was engaged to the love of my life, soaking up a broader way of seeing the world and my relationships in it, and I had become part of my family again, as well as Karen's. Not only that, but my back situation, though occasionally ornery, was dramatically improved.

Karen and I made good friends with our classmates at the healing school, and our social circle grew. We joined a nearby Catholic Church and got involved as lectors reading scriptures at the Sunday masses. I even Rolfed the pastor, the monsignor. We had gone to this particular church one Sunday because it had no steps, and my mother was on crutches from a spill on some ice. (Remember this was the winter of winters.) As I listened to the sermon, I knew I had found a kindred spirit in the monsignor. He was definitely preaching between the lines. When we met after mass, I learned he had gone to seminary with one of the (now married) readers from my dissertation committee. Such a tiny world. Karen and I felt instantly at home there.

We enjoyed the singing, the scriptures, and the community, and we tried to overlook the parts of the institutional Church with which we did not feel connected. We even choreographed a performance in word and movement of the Stations of the Cross during Lent. It was something I had done for the church I belonged to back in Chicago as well. For three years running at my parish there, I had been involved with and eventually took over the production of the Stations of the Cross. To intervals of music and scripture readings, myself as Jesus and fellow dancers in other roles would through movement render the story of Jesus' crucifixion. Since I was a "Tai Chi guy," I naturally performed the Tai Chi Jesus. People would stop me days after the performance to ask me how the heck I ever moved *so slowly*. It was a big hit, and touched people deeply.

Being back in New Jersey, I also reconnected with a woman whom I had known through volunteering at a grief support center years earlier. She had been one of the trainers. While I was off getting my Ph.D., she had embarked on a healing journey herself. After a trip with a shaman to the holy sites of Peru with her son and a friend, she spent five years studying with Barbara Brennan at her healing school on Long Island. Now we hit it off better than ever. Her son had been severely burned in a fire as a child. When I met him I instinctively began working my hands over his scars. It was as if his grafted skin fit him as a boy, but as a young man he had grown out of it. We soon set up a trade. I would Rolf her son and she would give healing sessions to Karen and me in exchange.

She was a source of relentless optimism and encouragement to me, and I came to treasure our visits, as did Karen. I was also hoping to support the healing that seemed to have begun to take hold in my back since the Rolfing training in Florida. We would sit facing each other and sort of work our way into a trance-like conversation. Eventually I would move to her healing table for "energy work." As we would sit, she would "open her vision" and see me in a greater light, while reporting what she saw. Oftentimes while looking at me in this state she would see my face and clothing change, flashing through a series of images of people I may have been, from her perspective, in past lifetimes, or perhaps just images of myself which were stored deeply within me. Invariably she saw monks and priests, gray robes and brown robes, cowls and beards, flashing by in series, with an occasional Buddhist or Taoist monk thrown in for good measure. It would seem I'd been working the "religious theme" for a good long time. I certainly felt that way. That was part of the delight of being with Karen "this time around." I was finally taking off those hoods and robes.

Not long before the upcoming performance of the Stations of the Cross, we went for a visit, and I told our healer friend what I was doing. I also incidentally mentioned my childhood "crucifixion" game. She looked me square in the eye and said, "So, you're *still* playing crucifixion?!" Her words struck me like a gong, and we both burst out laughing. We must have laughed for half an hour, that kind of contagious hysterical laughter that simply won't stop. Here was the counterpoint to the "mystical agony" I had endured in the Coffee Shop in Chicago that day. It was as if all at once I finally "got" the Cosmic Joke I had played on myself all of my life. Why the heck would anyone want to play crucifixion, over and over again? Why not play resurrection, or cards, for that matter?

Already for some years I had been a fan of the "Laughing Jesus." This was my practical counterpoint to the crucified Jesus. My aunt had sent me a picture of Jesus laughing which I had framed. He looked a little bit like Bob Marley, head back, in the throes of a good belly laugh. I even bought a sculpture of a laughing fish, which I kept next to this picture, the fish being an ancient symbol for Jesus. Our healer friend was a laughing Jesus fan too. She pointed me to a passage in the Gospel of Thomas, a text which circulated in early Christian times. In it, Jesus is said to have manifested at a distance in a cave, laughing and dancing with John, the beloved disciple, while everyone else is at the scene of the crucifixion weeping. Now, as I laughed with my friend, I understood with all my heart that I was meant for laughter, joy and resurrection, and that this business of playing crucifixion simply had to stop. As a student of Ida Rolf's teachings, I had learned that "gravity was the therapist." But as a student of Jesus, I wanted to be a student of levity and light, even in the midst of what seemed painful. Laughter is light, and a potent healer. It's no wonder Jesus laughed.

So this time, as I stood poised before the crowd with my arms outstretched, crying out my final agony and expiring on the cross, I just couldn't take myself too seriously, despite the kind ladies dabbing their eyes in the pews. In the past I would work myself into a froth of contrition and sorrow in preparation for "playing crucifixion." This time I set my heart on the truth of Easter and saw through the illusion of death. I just didn't feel like devoting my precious energy to making myself miserable anymore. I had a new litmus test for myself. In any given situation, did I find myself choosing to align with gravity or levity, death or resurrection? I knew what I wanted. That performance marked my permanent retirement from the role of Jesus dying, much to the disappointment of the pastor.

Having spent the last decade or so thinking about marriage, I may have had more well-formed opinions about what I wanted to express through the wedding liturgy than your average hubby-to-be, and Karen was very accommodating. We worked together to plan a ceremony that publicly marked our commitment and demonstrated our beliefs about marriage to the larger community. We got the monsignor to agree to hold the ceremony during the regular Sunday liturgy rather than at a time set apart from the regular gathering of the church community. We loved the passage from scripture where Jesus says, if you're going to have a wedding, invite people from the byroads, and not just your friends who can repay you. With our wedding open to anyone who happened through the door that Sunday morning, we felt we could fulfill that intent. We also passed over the more elaborate conventions regarding wedding costumes. I got a decent new suit fitting for any occasion, and Karen picked up a very lovely whitish dress at a second hand store about a week before the big day. Then early on in the ceremony, we had friends help us into identical white robes, something like baptismal gowns. The robes symbolized the "habit of love" to which we were publicly committing. I also felt if we started a trend, we could save poor couples the cultural obligation to spend their limited resources on elaborate wedding gowns if simple wedding robes were the "rage." No signs that we had any effect on that score. The elements of the marriage ceremony were woven into the mass, and the feeling with which we exchanged our vows were electric and palpable.

I can remember waking that day at around five in the morning. My buddy, the "dogma crusher," and my cousin of Euro-travel-partner fame were still pumping zees in the room we were sharing. I tiptoed out the door to sit by the brook on a swing and ponder the momentous occasion of our wedding day. Dew laden webs crisscrossed in the new morning's light, and I felt so happy to be weaving a life with Karen. I was also wired with the excitement of it all, friends and relatives swarming in for the occasion. With a several hour jump on the day, I had plenty of time to savor a moment of a day that sped past like a lightning bolt. Thank God the photographer insisted on getting a few garden shots of Karen and me at the reception, or we would barely have believed it happened.

We actually made the local paper, given the unusual nature of our ceremony. The reporter mistook our commitment to grow in our "habit of love" (the marriage) for the rest of our lives with a commitment to *wear* the "habit of love" (the wedding robes) for the rest of our lives. The paper made it sound like we would *never* take those silly things off. So much for witnessing to the masses. I can just see the Guinness Book of World Records now: "Couple sets record for continuous years in wedding clothes, and they are still going strong (and smelling strong too)." Our wedding day coincided with an after-church open social, so there were doughnuts and juice for the whole throng before family and friends headed over to a hall for a "smaller" party. We realized afterward that we had an average of 1.7 minutes to spend with each of the people who had populated our lives since childhood. So that ten minutes I spent helping a little boy in the potty eliminated a whole table of greetings! Weddings truly are whirlwinds.

We had planned a short honeymoon to Cape May on the Jersey Shore, with two weeks camping in Colorado to look forward to later in the summer. Nothing beats those first few days after a wedding, even if you've been living under the same roof. We were classic honeymooners, barely noticing the near hurricane force winds that punctuated our stay at the beach. We rode horses, toured the town, visited gardens, and ate romantic meals. Karen had begun working a couple of days a week in Philadelphia for a pregnant Rolfer friend. Since that was proving to be our most lucrative income stream at the time, we scheduled our little honeymoon around it, but in retrospect we would have gladly stretched our vacation longer. I never missed her more than when she drove off to Philly the day after our return from our time at the shore. I had a wife to miss! What a lucky fellow.

Now that we were married, Karen joined me in the attic until the downstairs tenants vacated the apartment which we were going to rent from my folks starting in August. With the healing school off for the summer, wedding booty counted, my practice picking up, my school loans not due for another six months, no more downtown office, and Karen bringing home the bucks from Philly, we started to feel a little better about our finances. When we flew out to Colorado in late summer for the annual meeting of the Rolf Institute and an extended camping trip, we had new hiking boots, a new tent and gear, and a new measure of self confidence.

Marriage was also proving kind to my back. Movement equals life, and we were moving together. Back in Chicago, I had enjoyed the foreshadowing that my commitment to becoming a Rolfer was a step towards incarnation. I enjoyed the life of the mind, but to the extent that I lived that life detached from my body, I wanted to change. I wanted to live my life inside my body, with love for my body, with a knowledge of it that was built on personal experience, and commitment to the goodness of my body. If Jesus incarnated, if spending a life in a body was good enough for him, then I wanted to commit to a positive relationship with my body as well. So long as I was alive in it, I had obviously had a relationship with my body, but it was a relationship that had been for the most part distant or hostile. Either I would ignore my body's needs, with irritation, or I would suffer it like some victim, enduring back pain as if my body were somehow "out to get me." By stepping away from the academic life and training as a Rolfer, I meant quite consciously to commit to the process of incarnation and to welcome it. I wanted to make friends with my body, to create a new relationship with it, to listen to what it had to offer me, rather than trying to just bully it into submission according to my will. My commitment to Karen and our relationship was another huge step in making conscious my "decision" to incarnate, to inhabit my body with kind purpose. Now it wasn't just *my* body, either. As her spouse, it was hers in a real sense too. By taking care of my own body better I was looking out for something that she valued dearly as well. I wanted to be in my body more because I enjoyed meeting Karen there, in the physical. It was an important part of our life together, and I knew I had to "own it" fully to share it fully.

Studying anatomy and working with clients were part of my "incarnation project" as well. Kind of like marriage, I figured if I was going to "take on my body," I wanted to study it and really come to understand it. But unlike my approach to marriage, where I had to justify the state in my mind before I was willing to experience it, I already had a body. The problem was, my experience of it was dissatisfying, and that's what I set out to improve. I wanted to figure out what the heck a body was, how it worked, what influenced my experience of my body, and how could I change that experience for the better. Out in Colorado at the annual meeting near Rocky Mountain national park, my expressed interests in anatomy provoked an invitation to the meeting of the anatomy faculty. At the meeting I suggested it might be a good idea to do a dissection together. Everyone loved the idea, and it was informally agreed that wherever someone came up with a cadaver first, the rest would meet there to do the dissection. I was excited, having wanted to explore dissection further ever since my experience back in Chicago.

Pending a dissection opportunity, Karen and I were excited to further our education in any way possible. On our return from Colorado, we took a five day workshop about working with the viscera, or guts, from a Rolfer in Manhattan. This guy was wired.

Never had I known anyone so excited about exploring the human body, and so capable of making that excitement contagious. Karen and I began to study with him in his office. He would work on Karen while I watched and asked questions, and then he would work on me while she observed. This fellow had actually gone to Barbara Brennan's school as well as having trained as a Rolfer, so we truly found a kindred spirit, given our own commitment to our healing school. Working with him, I experienced a level of connection in my body like I never had before. I couldn't hold the experience for very long, but it opened up in me an entirely new sense of what was possible for me. I knew that I could feel good in my body. He also challenged some of my perceptions about my body. He spoke as if even bones could be transformed through touch and movement, and I believed him. I stopped believing that my bones were some hard, unchangeable substrate of my body, and imagined that they were rubberized and could liquefy to re-form in ways that suited me better. I began to touch my clients with these beliefs and watched as marvelous changes took place before my eyes. I began consciously to reconceive my body.

Six months into our marriage, conceiving bodies one way or another was definitely on our agenda. Having moved into our own apartment downstairs, we were up visiting my folks one evening when my father looked at Karen and told her she was pregnant. This was the guy, you'll remember, who made his blood-oxygen readings bob up and down at will, so far be it from him to pick up on a thing like that out of the blue. We scoffed, chagrined, but he was right of course. Karen and I were open to having children, but hadn't put anything on a schedule, as it were. Our method of birth control was the infamous "calendar guess" method. That is, you look at each other, and guess that it *must* be a "safe" time of the month. Then you go for it. We assumed that the line of little beings hoping to get in on such a happy couple as ourselves was long, but we had no idea how *urgent* they all were. When the little line showed up on the home test kit, I was thrilled, and Karen was in shock. After shock, then thrilled. Now we really had a lot on the plate. Within a few months, Karen was showing, still nauseous, and still itching. My rather large loans came due, we were paying rent, the healing school tuition was piling up on the credit cards, our Rolfing practices were going but going slowly, and I was feeling a bit overwhelmed with the responsibilities which lay before me. Now it was my turn to be someone's father, and I must admit I was intimidated by the prospect. No sooner had I retooled my self-image sufficiently to see myself as a husband, and I had to retool all over again to see myself as a daddy. Golly, would things ever stop changing?

Karen and I studied up on birth and parenting with a vengeance. With hats off to our own parents for having pulled it off in their own way, we were determined to re-evaluate some of the choices surrounding pregnancy, birth and parenting which seemed obvious to our culture at large, but suspect to us. I had a chiropractor client who had mentioned on the table more than once his relief that his fiancée, like himself, did not believe automatically in childhood vaccinations. At the time, I thought he was crazy. I had never heard anyone question childhood vaccines before. Now that we were expecting a baby, I wanted to understand the basis of his concerns. He shared literature with me that made me realize the issue deserved intelligent consideration, rather than knee-jerk compliance to standard medical practice. Furthermore, I bridled at the notion that the laws appeared to mandate medical procedures and immunizations that had the potential to cause harm as well as good. From my study of medical ethics in school I was aware of the importance of free and informed consent to any medical procedure. Here, I found the law obliged procedures which definitively held the potential to harm my child, with various threats abounding for failure to comply. Where was the free and informed consent in that? It felt an awful lot more like coercion than consent to me.

The issue struck a nerve and I found myself obsessed and ranting about it like an angry child. It was the feeling of the popes all over again, except this time it was the medical establishment and the government telling me what was right and wrong, irrespective of my considered opinion, contrary knowledge, or cherished beliefs. With the popes I had taken on the belief that they had some special access to the meaning of scripture and the wisdom of the Holy Spirit, to which I must concede for my spiritual safety and well being. With the medical establishment and government I had taken on the belief that they had some special access to the means of health and the wisdom of science, to which I must concede for physical safety and well-being. Upon learning otherwise, my sense of betrayal ran deep in both instances, and I reacted with virulence. If I had taken steps towards maturity in my faith and an adult relationship with my parents, I was definitely starting from scratch when it came to the government and the medical establishment, whom I lumped together in a conspiratorial plot.

I was paying my storehouse of anger and fear a visit, this time in the guise of righteous parental indignation regarding the infringement of liberty and the health and safety of my yet to be born child. Threaten my baby, will you! For that I would fight to the death, forget writing some measly dissertation to figure it out. This one was going to take a bit of work. It was kind of like the flip-side of the "needing to be right/good" conundrum. There, for lack of an inner conviction of it, I felt compelled to prove my goodness by being right about this and that. Here, someone else (the government and medical establishment) who was supposed to be good was telling me I was wrong and therefore bad and unlawful when my inner conviction knew otherwise. And I was supposed to trust this leadership like a sheep, unquestioningly, even after I had discovered "the man behind the curtain." Now I not only took on the role of the innocent victim, feeling out of control, but with a little twist of paranoia: "they" are going to come and get me if I don't bend to their will.

So, I learned with joy and exhilaration that I was going to become a parent and not long after found myself waging a fearsome internal war between myself and generic "powers over me." Expansion, contraction. It must be in the script for life on planet

Earth. It is clearly in the script for *my* life on planet Earth. Thank goodness I am able to diversify my obsessions, or I would have gone mad. Six months had past since the anatomy faculty meeting. I called around to find out who had arranged for the group cadaver dissection, and found everyone basically scratching his head saying "cadaver, what cadaver?" I took the matter in my own hands and picked up the phone book. Within minutes I was speaking to the right person at a local university. Finally, becoming "Dr. Hedley" was paying off. I never pretended to be a medical doctor and didn't have to. I was a trained academic, and the field of anatomy is run by academics, not medical doctors. So we shared common ground. I wrote a proposal as a representative of the Rolf Institute's anatomy faculty that we would convene with the Department's permission in their laboratory to do a short-term cadaver dissection research project together. I went and met the inspiring gentleman who ran the laboratories. He gave me a thorough going over and we hit it off warmly. Before you knew it, I was calling back the anatomy faculty announcing the dates of our group dissection. I was thrilled that the doors had opened to the opportunity so quickly and easily.

But as the story is told in the Scriptures, a man sent his servant to invite friends to his wedding. The servant returns with their apologies, but no takers. "Sorry, I just bought a new field and I need to go stand in it." Such was my lot. Now I had two weeks scheduled with a cadaver in a university laboratory, no money to pay for it, and nobody to dissect it with me. This wasn't looking good. In the scripture, the groom sends his servant back out to basically shake people out of the bushes to come to his wedding since the invited guests turned him down. I decided to take the same approach. I started calling New York Rolfers, then New Jersey Rolfers, then Maryland Rolfers. "Hi, my name is Gil. Would you be interested in taking an experimental dissection workshop offered at cost?" I called until my little banquet was full, and leveraged the wealth of others to create an opportunity for myself as well as them.

Leverage is a basic principle which I was trying with enthusiasm to understand. In our healing school, our classmates ranged from starving artists to accomplished entrepreneurs to "old money." Placing myself in the category of starving artist, I felt lucky to know folks who had shed their robes of poverty long ago and learned how to be comfortable with wealth. Even though I was shedding those monastic robes with Karen's help, I felt like I was still encased in a virtual shell of poverty, and my bank account and credit cards proved it. On more than one occasion in my pious past I can remember having vowed myself to St. Francis's beloved "Lady Poverty." Now I wanted to shake her off like a bad smell, but our mutual attraction seemed old and intimate.

My body mirrored my bank account. Despite gains I had made in terms of my movement, I hadn't gained a pound in meat or fat since losing my body-builders mass dating that first college love thirteen years earlier. My body was what an anatomist would call transparent. My muscles and veins were all clearly visible. I had virtually no adipose layer, no reserves of stored fat, and I weighed the same as I did sophomore year in high school. Now some folks would consider this a situation to be envied, but I saw my lack of reserves in my body as a literal manifestation of my lack of reserves in the sphere of money. Have you ever seen a skinny king and queen?

Especially in light of my impending fatherhood, I decided it was time to commit myself to building a "reservoir." A reservoir became my symbol for the ability to build up a supply of something, in this case money. Perhaps I might even gain a few pounds. I had a conversation with wealthy friends from the school, who introduced me to the concept of leverage. She had made her money as a broker, he was raised with inherited wealth, and knew how to handle it. They both inspired me. When her clients made a dollar, she made a penny. Having had a lot of clients with a lot of dollars, she made quite a few pennies. The more they made, the more she made. She leveraged other people's money, putting it to work for herself as well. That, I thought, was profound.

Then a Rolfing client reiterated the theme abruptly one day. He was young, hefty, six foot three at least, and rolling in cash. At twenty-seven he was the country's largest manufacturer and distributor of body-piercing jewelry. That was quite a fad to be leading, and he did it by example. It was something of a challenge to work on him at times, actually, between the studs, rings and sundries, not to mention an array of entertaining tattoos to distract me as well. He came waddling in session after session, as one of his more inventive piercings was delayed in healing. And I was supposed to help his posture and fluidity of movement. Getting up from the table after a session one day, he announced, "Gil, the problem with being a Rolfer is that you don't have any leverage. You can only work on so many people, and if you're sick or they don't come, you make nothing at all. I have a whole factory full of people making money for me. You should just *hire* a bunch of Rolfers to work *for* you." Who was giving who a session here, I wondered. With that, he slapped his wad of cash in my hand, waddled out the door, and sped off on his Harley.

CHAPTER SEVEN

Models and Idols

Now I had leveraged other people to pay for the dissection, and I felt ingenious for that, but I still had placed no value on my contribution for having created the opportunity. I forfeited two weeks of paying work to lead the classes, but had charged the participants so little I barely covered the cost of tolls and lunch. Obviously I still had a lot to learn about leverage. Because I had already worked with cadavers to some small extent in the past, I was able to lead the group, but not without mustering all of the courage I had. Working with a whole cadaver from scratch was very different from picking up on someone else's work as I had done with my medical student friend back in Chicago. That had been challenging in itself. But I will never forget making that first untutored cut with my scalpel blade into a whole human form. There was an immensity to the act: I became an initiate into a fairly rare group of people. It's one thing to see a dead, embalmed human form. Anyone who has ever gone to a wake has experienced that, which in itself requires courage. It is an entirely different order of activity to take one of those forms apart by hand. I felt an immense gratitude for the woman who had donated her body for study. We repeatedly acknowledged the incredible privilege which we enjoyed in discovering and revealing the forms which fill our insides through her example. We also had a lot of fun, as cadavers are full of surprises, and the illusions we had generated for ourselves from our book-study of anatomy took a beating in the face of "the real thing." By the end of the two weeks, I was completely hooked on dissection, and determined to come back and do it again. I was also going to make sure I got paid for my efforts and experience the next time.

But that was a year away, it was now July, Karen was due in October, and my Rolfing practice was not nearly where it needed to be to support a family of three, much less pay the midwife's fee, however reasonable. Karen and I had made the decision to bypass the traditional route of medical birth in favor of a home birth. For one thing, we didn't have any health insurance and weren't really in a position to pay the extraordinary expense of a hospital birth. That was really not the most relevant consideration, however. We simply could not find an example in the animal kingdom, other than a Western Industrialized Human, who, upon going into labor would promptly leave its nest, expose itself to strangers, bright lights, and intrusive touch, and then relinquish the newborn to be handled by others and even kept at a distance to promote "rest." All the other creatures seemed to hunker down in the dark quiet warmth of the nest, give birth, remain in constant physical contact with the newborn, and bite chunks out of any pesky intruders. We decided the latter suited us better.

We also noticed that upon Karen beginning to show, total strangers would feel obliged to come up and retell in vivid detail the trauma they had endured during their labor. This seemed to provide some strange satisfaction to folks, as if somehow such warnings to the ignorant would serve to overcome our naivete and prepare us for the inevitable. We decided it was best to develop our own strategy. Rather than passively allowing ourselves to be surrounded by frightful and negative birth stories, we chose the opposite. We actively sought out people and books that reported beautiful and "unusually" smooth and glorious labors and childbirth scenarios. Our midwife reported a birth she had attended recently where after several hours of hard labor in the summer heat, the woman tired at about five centimeters of cervical dilation and decided to just take a break. Sitting for a couple of hours in a rocking chair, everyone thought she was napping. But then she opened her eyes and announced that the baby was coming out now, and without further ado proceeded to deliver her newborn. Apparently, she reported that she hadn't been sleeping at all, but rather meditating to open her cervix completely, and with great success. Now that was more our speed. We worried how our folks would take our decision, but it turned out Karen's dad had been born at home on a farm, and Karen's mom knew close family whose life had been saved by a midwife at birth. My folks were kind of tickled by the prospect as well, or at least deftly hid their concerns from us. We settled as quickly as possible into our plans to give birth to our baby without fear.

I redoubled my efforts to generate a busier practice, but the fact of the matter was, I could only manage a couple of clients a day. The work was hard, and as a relatively new practitioner I probably exerted more effort than was necessary. My back had improved from being Rolfed the second time, but actually making a living doing the work took a regular toll on my body, and it was all I could do to keep myself together while trying to help other people out.

Fortunately, one thing does have a way of leading to another. A friend of ours from the healing school had a little party to celebrate her newborn baby joining the world. At the party I began excitedly reporting my recent adventures in the anatomy lab to a woman from our class. She was so intrigued that she wanted to hear *everything* I had to say about anatomy, and suggested I put a course together to teach our other classmates. The healing school had an anatomy requirement, which basically amounted to the tedious project of coloring in all of the plates in the "Anatomy Coloring Book," nothing anyone particularly wanted to do. Perhaps, she felt, if I could teach a class, the assignment would be more palatable, or even unnecessary.

I let the idea stew for a while, and then I ate it up. I outlined twelve two-hour classes and set up a weekly evening at a friend's apartment in Manhattan. My class was invited to attend, and about ten people came. I charged a small tuition, but this class had no cadaver of course, so with the low overhead I actually made some money. And unlike Rolfing, the wear and tear on my body was minimal. I was back to studying and reporting on what I learned, but this time I was *getting* paid instead of paying to do it. Now *that* was exciting. Furthermore, it was the body I was studying this time, which fit right into my "project" to incarnate fully.

It has been said that if you really want to learn something, then teach it. I loved studying anatomy and physiology, especially having more dissection experience under my belt. The information seemed more meaningful now that I could relate it back to the cadaver I had just worked on. I marveled at the intricacies of physiological function. I was and remain consistently amazed at just how many millions of activities and processes are happening simultaneously beneath our conscious awareness to maintain our living human form. So many people get in a tizzy: "Everything went wrong today!" This because they were stuck in traffic or some such incident, unaware that countless numbers of specific physiological events happened with perfect success to maintain their bodies that very same day. The proportion of things going right to things going wrong on any given day are always trillions to one. That's good news.

As I thought about what I wanted to present in the evening classes, I realized I wanted to talk about the human body, yet I still couldn't even say for sure what the heck a human body was. What conception of the human body could summarize it adequately? I recognized the importance of how I described my body from my earlier struggle to say what marriage is. As mentioned, one of the major lessons of the dissertation was recognizing the relationship between what you call something and how you *behave* relative to it. How I conceive my body both describes and directs my relationship with it. Now I had spent a good portion of my life struggling with religious conceptions of my body, and in many ways I had shaped myself accordingly. My body was a pain in the ass, on that score.

There are probably hundreds of religious conceptions of the

body which could be described, but the ones that shaped me were of a certain variety. For instance, from the New Testament I heard St. Paul describe that there was a war being fought within "his members," one that seemed to get the best of him at times. To my very youthful mind, I knew *exactly* what he was talking about. My hormones kicked in indiscriminately at an early age, or so it seemed to me. As a sixth grader I can remember sitting in class with a raging "boner," as we called it back then. For no reason at all, my eleven-year-old body seemed capable of producing an erection instantaneously and without warning at the most inopportune times. I always left my shirts un-tucked to disguise my inevitable but stealthily hidden embarrassment. Is there anything worse than being called on to read your book report before the class while you have a flag raised which simply will not lower? Always be prepared. I suffered these indignities alone, never having had the matter explained, and assuming I was the only one with such a problem. Certainly my sister's were free of this curse. Anyway, stuck between my chair and the front of the room, immobilized with embarrassment, one of my little friends, Jewish by upbringing, looked me in the eye and said, "What's the matter, Hedley, you got somthin' to hide?" So much for my camouflage. I was dumbstruck that he clearly saw through me, but thrilled that he dared to cross the divide of silence. Notwithstanding the knowledge that my friend knew about "boners" and didn't seem to hold any negative judgments about the matter, I for my part saw the battle plans being laid already. It was me against my body. My body was an unruly embarrassment, needing to be tamed. There was a war within my members, and I was going to win it. My body, in a real sense, was an enemy, and it was my moral obligation to subdue it, control it, to make that boner go *down*!

It took a lot of fervent "Hail Mary" prayers to win a battle, but my body seemed to be winning the war. Sitting on the big yellow school bus for an hour every morning on the way to high school, with all of that jostling about, it was all I could do to "pray down the flag" before disembarking. In many ways I was starting to hate

my body, even as I sculpted it with weight training. I had also
discovered masturbation. Now there was a "Pandora's Box." I must
have ranked among the world's guiltiest teenagers. Once again,
one of my Jewish friends surprised me one day when he bragged
that he figured he was the first guy in our class to have figured out
how to "jerk." I couldn't believe it. Here was a guy bragging for
having accomplished the thing for which I most despised myself. I
envied him. Remembering the earlier incident, I became convinced
my Jewish friends were being raised to think that sexuality was a
normal thing, a bodily function, certainly not morally reprehen-
sible in principle. So what was my problem?

My jealousy was not enough to displace my own basic disposition towards my body, for which I was finding ample support in
my religious community. After all, I was taught that Jesus wasn't
married, his mother was a "perpetual" virgin, and that all of those
brother's and sister's of the Lord mentioned in the scriptures were
really just his cousins. Clearly sexuality was suspect, and the body
along with it. After all, how many hours had I spent staring at
Jesus' crucified body hanging before me in Church. Now there's a
strong image to model one's body-concept on. St. Paul's body
seemed to annoy the heck out of him. He encouraged follower's of
Christ to be like himself, presumably a sexually continent wid-
ower, and if you weren't married, you were better off to stay that
way. In college I learned about the great hero of the Church, St.
Augustine. Augustine may be most remembered as the Christian
defender of the goodness of the material creation against those
who rejected it, the Manicheans. Mani, a fourth century religious
teacher, led a sect of dualists. These folks believed that spirit was
good and the flesh evil. A spiritually accomplished person was one
who rejected the flesh and all of its trappings in search of the
spirit. They abstained from sex and marriage, and Augustine was a
former follower of Mani before his conversion to Christianity.

The problem was, the apple didn't fall too far from the tree.
Augustine actually never succeeded in following Mani's teachings
while he was a member of the sect. It seems he could never bring

himself to give up his love for his wife, with whom he had a son. She was technically his "concubine." They were not permitted to be "married" because of class differences, but for all intents and purposes, they had formed a "habit of love" and were married in practice if not in law. It took his conversion to Christianity to fulfill the practical implications of Mani's hatred of life in the physical body and rejection of the material creation as evil, even while he preached the opposite. That's because in light of his conversion, Augustine threw off his former life (meaning the concubine and the kid) and "sinful" ways (including his sex life) to become a celibate priest, and eventually a powerful bishop of the Church.

Like myself, Augustine related his struggles to control the "appetites" of his body to those of Paul. The body and all material creation may have been "good," technically speaking. God created the world in six days, and called it "very good." There was no way around that one. But you could be damn sure me and my illustrious "saintly" predecessors were going to show our bodies who's boss. The call to fill the earth *and subdue it* was ringing in our ears. The body is earth, and while it may be good, it must be subjugated to the spirit. The body may be good, but the spirit is better. Body and spirit are unequal participants in the goodness of creation, it would seem, and split hierarchically, with spirit on top and body on bottom.

Believe and practice that kind of thinking for a dozen centuries or so and we shouldn't be surprised to come upon the extreme treatment of the body which we find in St. Francis of Assisi. Francis would quell the upwellings of desire to marry and have children by rolling his naked body in the snow. And I thought I had problems. With the body designated as Brother Ass, it makes perfect sense that he gave it regular whippings to keep the beast in line. This kind of self-abuse was a commonplace of medieval monastic practice, but it really wasn't seen as self-abuse, because "the self" was not identified with the body. The body was an "other" which needed to be subjugated, like any other dumb and insolent creature, to the will of man.

By the time I was in college, my appetites for food and sex simply ranked among the annoying demands which Brother Ass placed upon me. If I couldn't control them, I would ignore them as distractions from my spiritual quest. I went through my entire college career without studying the human body in the slightest. It was out of my field of interest. Why would I want to explore something I basically just wanted to shut up? My model of the body, "the body as burden," was coherent with my religious affinities, and my body came to reflect that model: skinny, pale, and stiff. To add to this, my inability to ultimately control the demands of my body and the guilt I felt for fulfilling those demands left me feeling like a victim of my body. I finally had to eat to live, and when I refused to have sex with my girlfriends or myself, I ended up having "wet dreams" on a nightly basis instead. Leaving my shirt un-tucked just wasn't going to cover for that one. My body was going to do its thing whether I approved or not. I saw myself as a powerless victim, with my body tormenting me like a petty tyrant. I just wanted to be rid of the damn thing, whether the theologians told me it was good or not.

My movements were determined by this worldview as well. In spite of all my Tai Chi practice, when I got to the Rolf Institute pre-training I still moved like a cloistered monk: back relatively still, head bowed, eyes to the ground. For years I had worn sweaters with the hood up. I volunteered to have my movement analyzed by the class, and the teacher invited me to try walking with my eyes on the horizon. This was a remarkable moment for me. I realized how for an awfully long time I had been avoiding meeting anyone in the eyes as I moved about. I also recognized immediately that this was a choice. By keeping my eyes trained to the ground, I avoided "sinning" by looking at a woman with desire.

No wonder the beaches in Nice posed a dilemma. The effect of this chosen posture on my body was palpable. It stilled my movement. When I shifted my eyes to the horizon, I moved with greater ease and fluidity on the spot. It really was a simple matter. I could take more in, and make more connections. I had more options. I actually had more life. In training my eyes and shutting down my movement, I was in fact shutting down the way that my body would normally function. Here I was begging God for a new spine, and I wouldn't let go of the one I had. All this from my refusal to accept my own bodily inclinations, shored up with religious metaphors. I had had an idea about what my body was and how I should be, and I suddenly understood its ramifications. I immediately faced the choice of whether to accept the appetites of Brother Ass which might arise if I loosened my pattern of movement, or not. Or perhaps better still, I needed to reconcieve my body altogether, dropping the former image of my body as a burden to be subjugated and ruled, and replacing it with something new. But what would that new conception be? Like anything newly conceived, it would have to develop through many stages before it was fully formed.

Milling about in the history of my experience was another religious conception of my body which rarely held sway over what I have already described. The notion of the body as a temple of the Holy Spirit seemed extraordinary , but I only had an intellectual grasp of it, filing it under "nice ideas." It was the "body as burden" which characterized my experience and relationship with my body. Besides, conceiving of the body as a temple of the Holy Spirit could cut both ways, metaphorically speaking. On the down side, it could lead to all sorts of purity and pollution issues: if my body is a temple of the Spirit, I must be careful not to defile the temple, to keep it "clean" with all sorts of moral rules, etc. I had definitely used the "temple" model in that way in my pious "body as burden" phase.

On the other hand, if the body truly is a temple, a dwelling place of the Almighty, then its movements and attributes should be considered to reflect and manifest that very same animating life force of the Holy Spirit. Maybe God actually gave voice to great truths through the needs and desires of my body. In that case, I would do well to study my body very carefully, to understand its voice and listen for the word of God expressing itself to me, there in the temple. With this concept I realized that I had been sitting for my whole life outside the doorsteps of the most finely wrought Cathedral ever built, without ever having gotten off my arse to walk through the doors and have a look about. My body in all its complexity represented the wonders and workings of God's creation. Rather than being some insufferable obstacle to spiritual growth, my body as a temple of the Spirit could become my greatest resource for beholding the hidden face of the Divine within me. Now *that* motivated me to know God in a way that fasting, abstinence and the general betrayal of "Brother Ass" never had. I needed to get busy and learn my way around the inside of the breathtaking temple of the Spirit.

Of course, at this point I was not influenced by religious models of the body exclusively. Raised to be an upstanding, public-schooled U.S. citizen, my understanding of my body was heavily influenced by the dominant medical system of our culture as well. I learned the conventional scientific paradigms. I had been devouring scientific information about the body for years by the time I began teaching my anatomy classes. And in order to teach them well, I devoured all the more. However, now I knew there was such a thing as a "conception of the body" or "body concept" which invariably underlay any attempt to discuss, study or experience it. Any concept of the body carries with it a whole boat-load of assumptions which can be inspected and evaluated. The model with which I related to my body profoundly expressed and influenced my relationship with it. I dared to generalize my experience. Everyone is living their "bodily life," consciously or unconsciously, under the influence of some or several concepts of what they think their body *is*. That goes for biologists, physiologists and doctors as well as religious folks, agnostics and atheists. Animals in general or bacteria do not conceive of their bodies, except in the reproductive sense. If you have a body and a functioning mind, however, then you will unavoidably have developed a concept of your body which expresses and influences your experience of your body. And if you are not satisfied with your experience of your body, or want to change it just for fun, you would do well to make conscious your unconscious choices and assumptions regarding it.

My lifelong desire to "fix" or "get a replacement" for my back reveals how I had unconsciously adopted a mechanical conception of my body. On the mechanical model of the body, if something in my body isn't working, I just need to pay (or in my case, pray to) someone who knows about such matters to fix it. Quick fixes are definitely preferred. This is the model which prevails in science and medicine. Just pick up a physiology textbook. My favorite one proudly asserts from the start that the discovery and explanation of the mechanisms of bodily function is the main task at hand. No secrets there. The rules of the game basically state that the body is a machine, and that by studying the machine in great detail, taking it apart piece by piece, chemical reaction by chemical reaction, we can eventually figure out how it works. It's also no fair, according to this concept, to interject a non-mechanical explanation of how something might be working. Any non-mechanical explanation smells of "vitalism" or religion and "mysticism."

There do remain before the mechanist the disconcerting and unexplained facts that the "machine" of the human body is alive and self-conscious. These are conveniently reduced to self-contained mechanisms of the machine as well, because that is what mechanists do. You won't hear a die-hard mechanist wax eloquent about the power of the life energies moving in a living being, any more than you would hear someone who saw the body as a "beast of burden to be subjugated" sitting down for a pedicure and a facial. It ain't gonna happen. The person who views the body as machine nonetheless must confront these issues. When faced with the fact that the living human body draws breath about twenty thousand times a day from birth to the final expiration, the mechanist speaks of "a self-sustaining oscillator" located in the brainstem. Medulla oblongata plays *deus ex machina*. The same play is made for the continuity of the heartbeat over a lifetime, one hundred thousand times a day. The heart is said to be "autorythmic." Find me a car with perpetual air intakes, pistons that fire themselves, and hun-

ger pangs for gasoline, and I'll show you a human body that is
adequately characterized as a machine.

The problem with models of the body, or any model, for that
matter, is that they are only effective in revealing a partial truth by
means of purposely excluding the whole truth. Models reduce reality. They reduce them to tiny bits and pieces that our developing intellects can digest. Because our rational intellects have certain limits, we grasp at models. They are by definition partial rep-
resentations of the truth. The simplest line drawing was sufficient
to teach my daughter to recognize a horse. And with a little whin-
nying at the picture on my part, I was thrilled to hear her whinny-
ing from her car-seat at the real horse grazing in the pasture as we
drove by it. Models can point to more full realities. They are never
the whole truth. A toy choo-choo is not a commuter train. Just try
riding one to work. I also would be foolish to argue that a horse
must have only the properties and characteristics of a two dimen-
sional line drawing, because that's where I learned about horses.
As surely as a model can point to more full realities, it is a mistake
to believe that the reality is ever sufficiently portrayed by the model.
While it may be incredibly instructive and productive of insight
to conceive of the body as a machine, to insist that it is or can be
nothing but a machine mistakes the model for the reality.

I had a housemate and dear friend in Chicago who was an
economist. She subscribed to the "rational actor" model of the
person, which basically presumed that all human actions were con-
trived to attain the self-interest of the person acting. Basically, all
motives were presumed selfish, and from that, certain general be-
haviors in the marketplace and other spheres of life were predicted.
Now Milton Friedman, the beloved grandfather of Chicago-style
economics, never presumed that the "rational actor" model sufficiently described all human behavior. He knew such a reduced
portrayal of human motivation was simply a generalized tool with
which to prod the earth of the economy. But this pupil who had
descended from that lineage had come to believe that the model
was the whole truth. Her interactions with my other housemates

repeatedly revealed her suspicion of their motives, based on her particular economic model of the person. Needless to say, she didn't get along with many of the fifteen people in the house. Everyone was presumed selfish, and out for their own interest exclusively. She was truly a dear person herself, but her model skewed her experiences a bit. If someone appeared altruistic, it was safe for her to assume that underneath the appearance lay selfish motives still. There was nothing that could convince her otherwise, because she only permitted herself to consider people in light of the rules of her singularly reductive model.

I wrestled with so called "Creationists" at Duke who demonstrated a similarly closed circle of reasoning. Certain "fundamentalist Christian" acquaintances who were attempting to convert me from my Catholic ways would engage me in arguments for their "biblical" account of God's creation of the world. Their claims were made in adherence to a "literal" account of creation based "on the Bible alone," which for them seemed to be the sole source of truth on the subject. Therefore, they claimed the earth was a total of five thousand and some-odd years old, along with a host of other "biblical facts." I introduced in response the accomplishments that had been achieved with carbon-dating, or pointed to the fossil record, or the geological history represented by the visible strata of a formation like the Grand Canyon. They replied from within the limits of their conception of creation: "Since God created everything, surely he could create fossils too, or make the Grand Canyon look as old as he wanted." This was obviously a conclusive argument from their perspective. In fact, it was merely circular. It was coherent with the rules of their model, or conception of creation. But it was incoherent with the signs within nature which might illuminate the truth of God in a different way than the language of scripture.

Like the mechanist who will only permit internal mechanisms (or, with limits, the physical forces of the environment) to explain bodily functions, or the economist who will only permit a singular characterization of human motivation, the creationist has reduced permitted descriptions of the physical world to their so-called "literal" interpretation of the Bible. In each of these cases, the partial truth of the model is mistaken for the whole truth to which it points. It is one thing to believe that the material universe is created from the Divine mind and word, and quite another to insist it must happen according to one descriptive and humanly comprehensible timeline. It is one thing to recognize the selfish motives of human behavior, and quite another to act as if selfishness is the exclusive possibility. And finally, it is one thing to explore thoroughly the very real and remarkable physical mechanisms of the human body, and quite another to reject out-of-hand the emotional, mental, spiritual and relational realities which might enhance our understanding of bodily functions.

Once I recognized the power of the assumptions underlying my own conception of my body, I became more adept at grasping the truths pointed to by other models without falling for the model as the whole truth. After all, mistaking the model for the truth is the very basis of idolatry, as I understand it. I was tired of falling for the idols I had set up for myself, believing that my body was just a burden or some broken machine needing a tune up. I wanted more from my experience of living life in a body than I could have from within the limits of my past conceptions. Crafting my body into the "ultimate machine" with weightlifting created distortions in my structure from which I am still healing. Treating my body like a stubborn mule resulted in many years of self-imposed frustration and misery. Acknowledging my body as a temple of the Spirit definitely put me on a different track, allowing me to reconceive my body for the better. In attempting to explore with my little start-up anatomy class some sort of answer to the befuddling question, "What is a body," I found myself firmly on the path of reconceiving my own body, not just once, but over and over again. By dropping the rules of what I permitted myself to believe about my body, I began to see and experience myself in new ways.

CHAPTER EIGHT

Unwrapping the Heart of Pleasure

After teaching the class for about four weeks, I had to cancel the following lesson. Coming down the stairs to our apartment from the office after doing two Rolfing sessions the day before Halloween in 1995, I saw a look on Karen's face that could only mean one thing. Here comes the baby! Karen awoke that morning noticing the little "preview" contractions were picking up the pace, and had gone out to do some errands. She reported that the contractions started to hit hard on line at K-Mart. Attention, shoppers! Would the lady in aisle three please have your baby somewhere else! I had heard about the shift in a woman's focus as she goes into serious labor. I could see Karen was already dropping in for the duration. I called for the midwife, cancelled that night's class, and started filling the portable hot tub we had set up in our living-room-bedroom-dining-room. Many folks think that a "water birth" is especially good for babies, which may be so, but we set it up primarily for Karen. The warm water was soothing and made her pregnant body lighter while she focused on the delivery.

The midwife and her assistant arrived with about an hour to go. The room was candlelit, and Karen embodied the living archetype of the Mother Goddess. The air in the apartment was thick with the ancient rite of birth, and it seemed as if, though there were only four of us present to the eye, the room was crowded with what felt like a host of Native Americans, "old friends" of Karen's, all supporting us in the unfolding of this electrifying process. I watched with amazement and awe as my beloved wife took to delivering our baby as if she had done it a thousand times, with extreme intent of purpose and courage. She was awesome. As she knelt in the tub facing me, I saw the bones of her pelvis with potent vibration literally float apart as she pushed the baby through. I climbed in to support her for the final passage. The midwife scooped the little one from the water into Karen's arms, and we, now three, floated there together, weeping with delight and gratitude. It was all we could do to repeat aloud our thanks to God over and over again while we marveled at this little being squirming in our midst. She began nursing almost immediately, and we gently climbed out of the water and into the bed. After about an hour of this, we finally drew back the blanket. It hadn't occurred to any of us to see what sex the baby was, so entranced we were by the fact that there had *really and truly* been a baby in there after all. This honestly came as a shock! It took us another week to give her a name. We were in no rush, and figured we'd get to know her before naming her for life. We finally arrived at Sarah, for the mother of Isaac and wife of Abraham, who laughed out loud at the angel upon hearing she would bear a child. Her middle name is Grace, to remember our overwhelming gratitude for her having come to join us and make a family of us.

We didn't answer the phone for nearly a month, and four years later we still haven't sent out birth announcements. Such is our pace about these things. Within two hours of Sarah's arrival, the midwives departed out the door with their tub in tow, and we were snuggling in the glow of new birth. I was amazed at how comfortable I felt handling her. I had never felt so confident with my sister's babies as I did now with my own. My parents came home after having been consigned to wander the mall for the day, and they concurred that the house felt really good, washed in blessing. My mom had warned me that I simply would not believe how much I could love my own child, and now I knew what she was talking about. My ability to love had increased exponentially on the spot. Our life has never been the same. That's actually how we know it's our *life*. Stasis, failure or refusal to move, change and grow, is the formula for a rut, and ruts pre-form graves. Kids have kept me moving faster than I ever believed I could, and I still feel like a slug compared to them.

Upon becoming a father and seeing my wife and precious daughter lying there looking so vulnerable, I definitely felt a wave of responsibility which must be familiar to fathers throughout the ages as well. Not a bad feeling, just a feeling: time to go out and slay some buffalo. But I also found myself living in a most marvelous classroom, with Sarah Grace Hedley as my new teacher. Frankly, the draw to her outweighed the call of the buffalo by a hefty margin, and I was happy to be making my living mostly out of our home. Now here was a body to behold. Watching Sarah as a baby, I was able to witness human movements free of any overlaying conception at all. It was not that she moved with her body effortlessly. Babies are forever jerking and pawing and straining for this and that. Rather, she moved as a whole. Every movement was a movement of her whole body. When she went for Karen's breast, her whole being supported that suckling mouth. When she was startled, every limb was surprised from her very center. She clearly had no sense of time, or judgment, or even separateness from her mother. She was motivated rather from the sensations generated from within her body, and by her interaction with the sights, sounds, and touches from the people and things surrounding her.

It is odd that at least a generation or two in our country were conditioned to believe that the cry of a baby comes from its intention to manipulate its parents, who must quickly learn to show the baby "who's boss." There is truth in the notion that the baby manipulates its environment with its cry, but there is certainly no fathomable underlying intent to control or rule on the baby's part. That is a purely "adult" (mis)perception and projection. A baby experiences discomfort and it cries, because that is an outward expression in response to an unpleasant internal sensation. If the need for food or warmth is met, a healthy feedback loop is established between the baby's cry and the parents' response. If the cry is ignored, the loop of satisfaction is not established. The baby will continue to feel the sensations of discomfort nonetheless, but may need to establish other responses, such as holding or contracting to squelch the sensation, developing a tense musculature. Or a baby might simply "exit" its body to avoid the discomfort. How many people have said, "Oh, my baby cried for just a moment after the shot/circumcision, and then fell fast asleep. He was fine, no problem." Actually, sleep is an escape route from pain for a baby, though sleep is not always easily achieved. Have you ever seen a baby cry and sleep simultaneously?

Karen and I felt that with Sarah's birth we had really joined a new club. We had a deeper understanding and appreciation of our parents, in the first place. We now knew the details of all they had done for us without thanks or expectation. We also could look at other couples strolling their babies with insider knowledge of what their life was like, and we developed new friends in the neighborhood quickly. We had studied and believed strongly in the importance of ample bodily contact with infants as a wise "insurance policy" for their health and comfort. We carried Sarah constantly, even when she slept during the day. I learned how to peel oranges with one hand. Along the same lines, we kept a "family bed" at night. I was initially worried about sleeping with a baby, as most people in a culture where this is uncommon often are. For the majority of the world, it's standard practice. Most people don't even have the "luxury" to do otherwise, consigned to single-room homes as they are. I learned that family sleeping practices had altered considerably in this country from a hundred years ago. The protestant moralizers of the nineteenth century who roamed the country preaching in tents had considered the practice unseemly and it fell into disrepute here. However, my misgivings fell by the wayside the very first night. When sleeping-Karen leaned even slightly towards sleeping-Sarah Grace, Sarah reflexively alerted Karen with her arms and legs, and Karen would adjust accordingly. I witnessed what must have been eons in the making, the normal interactions of sleeping bodies, mother and child. The safety issue had been worked out long, long ago. In fact, I recognized the profound safety advantages of sleeping together for monitoring the baby's well-being. The arrangement also made nursing in the nighttime a simple matter. After a few days, I could no longer imagine *not* having Sarah with us.

While I observed the "organic" quality of Sarah's movement, the integration of her whole body with what she desired, it was not until I took a workshop some months later that I began to understand her experience more deeply for myself. I attended a five-day class sponsored by our healing school with a mover/healer/shamaness named Emily Conrad. In an article I later wrote about the experience for *Rolf Lines: The Journal of the Rolf Institute*, I coined the word *somanaut* to describe her. Like an astronaut who navigates outer-space, a somanaut is a person who navigates the inner-space of the body. Emily was the ultimate somanaut.

I had heard about her for some time, and was anxious to learn from her insights about life in human form. She called her work Continuum. The basis of her deep exploration of the body was rooted in personal experience. For many years, she had experimented with breath and movement, especially internal movements provoked by different types of breath exercises. She would teach a certain kind of breathing exercise, and then encourage her students to follow and yield to the internal sensations and movements which arose in their bodies as a result of the particular breath. She didn't do it for you. Self responsibility is a hallmark of this work. Unlike forms of "treatment" which are structured around and subject to the dynamics of doctor-patient, Rolfer-client relationships, Continuum is something done alone or in groups, but it is wholly self-motivated. No one "does it to you," who can later be blamed for lack of success or put on a pedestal for achieving a positive outcome. There is no one to look to but oneself.

Emily was especially keen to point out that over the course of a lifetime, from conception to death, human beings assumed a great many forms. These forms ranged from the one-celled creature of the new conceptus, to the sometimes tadpole or fishlike embryo, to the hair-covered ape-like fetus, and so on. She further believed that when we are deeply connected to and exploring our physical bodies, it is possible to experience the range of sensations which are particular to any of those forms. They belong to our history but also our present, and are accessible. Watching her contact those places in herself was most compelling. Emily did not imitate a lizard. She exposed the lizard within. Emily also felt that what is considered "normal feeling" in our bodies more accurately represents the slow but progressive atrophying of sensation and movement over the course of a lifetime. We tend over time to progressively limit the range of sensations and movements which we permit ourselves, eventually freezing up the incredible range of sensations which are our birthright, and which we knew as babies. In her view, for the most part we are consistently limiting our nervous system and our bodily experience to a narrow rut. We pop the toaster, we turn the doorknob, we sit at the computer, we drive the car, we watch the tube. We hook into exercise machines at the gym which "strengthen" us according to the limited pattern of movement which the machine permits, rather than expanding us into the infinitely complex range of movements which our bodies have the potential to express. The intent of her breath and movement work is to break up the patterned ruts which our life-limiting choices have placed upon our movement and our bodily experience. By moving in ways unusual to our patterning, we feed our nervous system variety, and open new worlds of sensation and intelligence for ourselves.

Her work corroborated both the history of my own experience as I've described it, and also an experiment I conducted back in Chicago. Immediately after completing my dissertation, I decided to take a little vacation from the way I had been doing things in the past. For two weeks, everything for which I had normally used my right hand, I used my left, and vice-versa. I found myself brushing my teeth about five times more slowly, but with careful deliberation. Simply by holding the broom at the Coffee Shop opposite to my normal pattern, I found myself sweeping the whole place in reverse, and came across dirt I'd been missing for who knows how long. I got on and off my bicycle from the opposite side and opened the door to my apartment building otherwise. That turned out to be a much easier way to get through with the bike, something the local lefties must have taken for granted, I realized. I was amazed at how differently I experienced my day to day world upon making that simple change. I had also challenged my nervous system to learn new things.

Emily had raised challenging the nervous system to a fine art, and it was clear how her work held promise as a self-healing tool as well. At the workshop was a woman paralyzed a dozen years earlier in a car accident. After eleven years of physical therapy, she had achieved much for herself, but did not regain use of her legs. For Emily, by returning to those states of sensation from our formative period, we can tap and restore in ourselves as well the generative properties whereby we grew our body in the first place. If we grew a nervous system once, why not grow one again? This brings reconceiving the body to a very practical level. By finding and exploring what movement is available, one's range of sensation and movement can be fanned like a flame and spread to areas of the body cut off or previously excluded from sensation for whatever reason. Practicing the techniques of Continuum, this woman within two years had begun to restore sensation and movement in her legs, and was capable of crawling movements by the time of our workshop.

Belief most certainly plays a huge part in such an achievement. If one believed that it was impossible to restore sensation and movement from paralysis from injury, why bother trying? For all of the years I have been studying the "facts of science," textbooks have consistently presented the conclusive case that at a certain point in development, one's full complement of cells in the central nervous system is fixed. Therefore, if brain cells die off, tough luck. They are irreplaceable, as no new cells form there. That "fact" kind of puts the kibosh on hopes for the brain injured by way of restorative growth of nerve tissue. Yet recently it was announced in the press that experimenters had successfully demonstrated new cell production as a matter of course in a particular area of the adult human brain, with reasonable speculation of a more far-reaching phenomenon. The article also reported the skepticism with which the discovery was met. It flew in the face of "established" facts, and science resists a change like my wet-diapered son, kicking and twisting all the way. But reconceiving beliefs about the body could open doors to the discovery of new "facts" and the overthrow of previous ones based on more limiting concepts. Those creative scientists first had to be open to the very contrary idea that the brain might grow new cells before pursuing research to demonstrate it to be so. And having done so, they have opened the door to a flood of new creative questions regarding how we might foster and enhance that capacity where there is need. What other powers of body, mind and spirit functioning in union can I dare to imagine if I am willing to reconceive my body?

At the time of the workshop, I dared to imagine that I could improve the condition of my back. I was, however, admittedly frustrated three days into the class. My ability to discriminate the kinds of fine sensations which Emily and other people in the class described was limited. For all of my studies, I was still very "head centered," though I was toying with the borders of self-limitation. The sensations I was most typically aware of in my body were different types of pain. Over the years I had become sort of a "connoisseur" of back pain, and considered myself to be doing great when I couldn't feel anything at all. Consequently, what I felt on my forth day of breathing and subtle wiggling took me by surprise completely. I felt pleasure. It was a deep sense of pleasure that I felt, stirring in the heart of my upper back, previously the locus of so much misery.

I was able to stay with it for a short while, though given the novelty of the experience it seemed like a long time to me. Later I found I could return to the pleasurable sensation if I set my intent gently upon that. I marveled that it was repeatable. So pleasure was not just a fluke after all. I could choose to "go there" or not. Now you would think that such a choice was an obvious one, but

I can't say I immediately opted to perpetually enjoy pleasure over pain or numbness on the spot. Nearly simultaneous to my discovery that I could choose pleasure over pain, I learned something else about myself. I actually had a fairly limited tolerance for pleasure as compared to my huge tolerance for pain. My personal history was replete with choices for pain over pleasure, as I have recounted. It was almost as if in the world I had built for myself, I had placed a premium on pain and suffering, whereas pleasure was generally suspect. Despite my happy marriage and progress in accepting sexuality as an integral part of me as a person, the negative judgments I had held for so long about the pleasures of sexual expression had in a very real sense left their legacy in my body. To overcome my old judgments and conditioning, I had to do more than intellectually grasp the problem and believe something else about it. I had to be willing to practice "enduring" positive and pleasurable conditions and states in my body to build up a tolerance for them and displace the "comfort level" which I had achieved with pain and numbness. It was as if bodily pleasure in general had suffered from "guilt by association" with sex. The good news was, if sex could be redeemed, then so could pleasure in general, even in my back.

The culture of my religious heritage had elevated suffering to great heights. Suffering borne heroically could put one in the company of the saints and martyrs, who modeled themselves on Jesus himself. Or at least a certain version of him. How many times had I heard of so and so who "bore their suffering without complaint." According to this sort of logic, the greater your suffering, and the quieter you are about it, the more like Jesus you will be. I simply took my stand in a two-millennia-long line of people who have modeled their experience of their body on Jesus' death, rather than on his life and resurrection. Playing crucifixion was an old game, without much originality on my part. Where I had seen the choice at a certain level and laughed over it in the past, now I was experiencing the roots of it in my body and bringing to consciousness the unacknowledged choices I myself had made over and over again for pain. I really could choose pleasure instead. The living and risen version of Jesus, who himself understood and enjoyed the pleasures of bodily form, would not be offended.

Rather than representing the horror wrought by injustice, fear and ignorance, the model of Jesus' body crucified had somehow been transformed and mistaken, in my opinion, for a "good thing" in itself. The suffering servant, the lamb led to slaughter, the innocent victim all become models of sanctity by association. Therefore suffering itself becomes a legitimate path, zealously sought out by the venerated martyrs of the church: a veritable shortcut to heaven. The status of victim is exalted and linked with innocence, and innocence with holiness. So if I suffer some illness in my body and bear it stoically, I am "Christlike."

The distortions inherent here did not always appear obvious to me. I had long identified with the suffering servant. Enduring years of pain, I played the victim, never aware that I was unconsciously choosing my part on stage with the company of the "saints and martyrs." By keeping fairly quiet about my suffering, I upped the ante on its holiness-value. With this model, I conceptually split the self with which I identified off from my body. I was the victim, and my body the perpetrator. My back is killing me! I was innocent, and my body was guilty and endlessly guilt-provoking. I wanted to get out of my body, as if I were some little forest animal and my body a trap which I had stumbled upon, ensnaring me.

In this, my religiously formulated body concepts, whether "body as burden" or "body as perpetrator" or "cause of suffering," were united. In each formulation I created an essential separation of body and self. I am this spirit thing over here, and my body is this physical thing in which and with which my spirit must wrestle. Coming from a conception of the body as separate from the spirit, the union of the two seems forced, uncomfortable, and even dangerous to the spirit. Much like the Manichees against whom Augustine had railed, I had for the most part been a "dualist Christian," a walking oxymoron. No wonder I found St. Augustine so annoying. We had a lot in common. We both insisted the body was good but didn't "walk the talk."

So within the heart of pleasure in my back lay a "Pandora's Box" of insight and sensation for me. But I didn't practice Continuum for long. Instead, I simply filed the knowledge for myself that pleasure was available to me, something I could come back to when I had the time. I was glad to know it with deeper confidence. That is about what I was ready for at the time. But I was a busy daddy now, busy worrying about important things, like *money*. Money, money, money. I had started up a second little anatomy class for the healing school running concurrently with the first, and made a few pennies there. I was Rolfing several clients a week, though I never really had a full practice. What I really wanted was to put that principle of leverage I had been pondering into action. I wanted to crack through my "poverty shell" and vault my little family to financial prosperity. My parents had sent away for a home-training course on investing in the commodities markets. Gotta love those pork bellies. As a child, there were always little pamphlets lying around our house with titles like "Become Rich in Your Spare Time by starting Your Very Own Worm Farm." I devoured the course, seeing dollar signs lighting my way to the business section of the newspaper. All sorts of charts began to clutter our apartment. My dad put the lion's share of some money into an account with me which I planned to trade up into a fortune for us all.

Plugging me into the world financial markets and commodities futures was like putting a jackrabbit on intravenous caffeine. I rode the prices of corn, copper and Swiss Francs like a wannabee cowboy on a real wild bronco. I got thrown and trampled, fulfilling the prophecy of a friend and experienced businessman very quickly. He had said that "the surest way to make a small fortune in the commodities market was to start out with a larger one." I lost us a couple of thousand dollars, trading on pure emotion, one by one ignoring every rule the little course taught. Dad was chagrined but took his loss nobly. I learned that I could make money on paper easily and for real with difficulty. I simply lacked at that time the kind of maturity, discipline and emotional detachment necessary to trade futures effectively. I also wasn't ready to fill a reservoir when I had only built a puddle.

Therefore, what I did take from the course was the importance of saving a percentage of my income to build up my resources, regardless of what I owed. My tendency was that whenever I got some extra cash, I would immediately put it towards reducing some debt. In this way, I never saved a dime, and never had any reservoir. For years I had tithed to the Church and other charitable organizations ten percent of my income. This was simple enough when I was living off of student loans, giving away what was essentially someone else's money, while my expenses were minimal. Karen and I wanted to tithe and quickly found there wasn't enough money left to pay the bills, and our credit card debt mounted ever higher. We decided to put ten percent of our income into savings for a while instead and see what happened. Seeing ten and twenty dollar deposits slowly add up to a few hundred dollars was incredibly satisfying, and the lenders to whom we owed money didn't seem worse off. We may have saved tiny amounts by some standards, but it was a start.

In setting up another round of dissections for the summer, I learned that it was possible for me to leverage small past experience into larger future ones, without putting up a dime. That was more my speed. Having started a good relationship with the folks at the school where I taught the first year, I was able to expand the opportunity. This time I set up my schedule to spend a whole month in the lab: the first two weeks with some friends as a research project, and two weeks of teaching. I also charged my students a reasonable workshop fee to pay me as a teacher as well as to cover my costs for producing the class. I wasn't making a killing, but I did nearly cover the loss of my Rolfing practice for a month. It seemed like a fair trade. I was excited to get back into the lab.

This time, however, I was determined to do things differently. I felt that my approach was haphazard the year before, with minimal structure to the proceedings and little focus of direction. More importantly, I wanted to do dissection in a way that was coherent with my evolving sense and experience of my body as an integrated whole. The medical tradition of dissection is generally based on what is called "regional anatomy." The focus is on the part, not the whole. There is a real degree of practicality to this. Although a cadaver is an embalmed dead human body by definition, the state of preservation is not indefinite. When working on a cadaver over a period of time, one or two semesters, as medical students do, one must take good care to see that the cadaver lasts in a well preserved state as long as possible. Therefore it makes sense to work on a small exposed area thoroughly, before moving on to another region and exposing more tissue to the effects of the air. The medical student learns anatomy part by part, region by region. My first dissection experiences followed in this tradition. But there was more to the practice of regional anatomy than the admittedly important practicalities described. Underneath it lies certain assumptions rooted in the mechanistic model of the body. The process of learning anatomy by regions and parts is in fact an indoctrination. Whether consciously or not, the standard courses of anatomy seem to give practical substantiation to the belief that the body is in fact a machine built of discrete parts. An exquisite machine, it is conceded, but a machine nonetheless. Its parts can be differentiated, removed or even replaced. And because the model seems generally effective in practice, it is usually taken for granted to be true.

As a self-directed explorer, working in but not beholden to a medical educational setting, I enjoyed a freedom in my study of anatomy unknown to medical students. Those men and women who take up the long hard road to professional competence as doctors are under tremendous pressure to absorb the huge amounts of information before them. They are not really invited or given the time for much "free thinking" about the subjects at hand. They need to pass the test and move on to the next one, not ponder the underlying assumptions of what they are being taught. That's for the philosophers two buildings over. Having that freedom to explore other options and the condensed time frame of a six-day intensive workshop, I took another path. After all, my experience as a Rolfer, my observations of my daughter, and my growing experience of my own body had created a shift in my perception. I had become more prone to focus on the connections, the relationships and the wholeness inherent in the human body than on the separation of the parts. If I had become suspicious of models of my body which split it off from my spirit, I also grew uncomfortable with models of my body which divided it up in separate discrete little named pieces without deference to or appreciation of its unity.

But anatomy literally means to cut up with a knife. The named "parts" of the body were seen as different by those original anatomists because it was possible to separate them by passing a blade between them. And perhaps it's just plain trickier to grasp the whole than the part. Who can say? For having begun to reconceive my body, now I was going to have to reconceive anatomy as well. I wanted to teach and understand *integral anatomy*. If I was going to take something else apart, I wanted to do it with the intention of putting myself back together. Some years back there was a fad of posters which at first glance appeared to be just a wash of color. If you stared at the image long enough, and with soft enough eyes, the whole thing would shift and you would suddenly see an image of a tiger or a whale or some such thing. It was there all along, but lost to the first impression. Although for all the times I stared at those pictures I never managed to see the underlying image, I had much better luck with the body. My underlying hope for integral anatomy became two-fold. First, I wanted to support the shift of my perception from the part to the whole. Second, I wanted to increase my sense of internal connection through exploring the connections and relationships revealed in the human forms I studied, my own most importantly.

I spent the first two weeks in the lab that summer working out the practical details of "integral anatomy" for cadaver dissection. When we broke for lunch, I would steal off to call the commodities brokerage to check on corn and Swiss Francs. Wee little me was still trying to leverage the world financial markets at the time. Abandoning the regional approach altogether, we attempted to dissect the whole body one major layer at a time: skin, superficial fascia, deep fascia, muscles, organs, and bones. It proved to be a very powerful approach, which I immediately refined and repeated with the two classes which followed. By focusing considerable time and the attention of the whole group on a particular layer, we found ourselves appreciating the continuities and connections of whole layers, as well as understanding more deeply the relationships between layers. We also found ourselves feeling and noticing our particular reactions to the layer we were focused on, both physically and emotionally. By taking the time to "unwrap" the donor gifts one layer at a time, we began to discover and create relationships within the hidden layers of our selves.

CHAPTER NINE

Victims, Saviors, and Perpetrators

Needless to say, that summer in the lab was profoundly moving for myself and the groups with which I worked. I knew that I had created an opportunity for self-discovery through anatomical exploration which was unique and potentially even life-changing. Unfortunately I coughed for two months straight after having spent four solid weeks breathing cadaver fumes. I was going to have to take better care of myself if I was to continue to do this work for my own sake, no less generate some extra income with it. My Rolfing practice was small in the first place, but putting it on hold for a month nearly fried it altogether. My forays in the market were failures in general. Just when I was about to make some money I would panic and sell, making a few dollars or preventing a loss, but mostly just wasting my time. By summer's end, despite all the good things in my life, my precious daughter, loving wife and good family relations, I was depressed. What few Rolfing clients I worked on left me in worse shape than they. I had demonstrated my incompetence at trading. I had periodically followed the academic teaching market in my field, which was very tight. Despite the fact that I had no desire to teach in academia, I would apply for jobs anyway. Those applications invariably fell flat. I had removed myself from the circles of influence which might have landed me a job, and I didn't really want one anyway. We had spent three years in our healing school and had borrowed the tuition for both of us, so now we were in debt to the extreme between that, our Rolfing training, our failed office fiasco, and my Ph.D. I had a bad case of feeling like I had learned a lot and was accomplishing nothing.

I turned to the newspapers, thinking perhaps I could find a "normal" job and at least have a reliable income to support my family. I even nosed around my old garbage hauling buddies, without giving any indication I was thinking about a job. They were fully staffed with reliable help, I learned. And what's up with you? Oh well. When I called up to make inquiries on newspaper ads, folks would literally laugh at me. It seems my Ph.D. overqualified me for just about anything I saw in the paper, despite garbage truck driving having been the only full-time job on my resume. I felt like I kept trying to walk through shut doors. But this was no dream, and I was bumping up against myself. Finally in desperation I went to fill out an application at a local limousine service that was looking for drivers. I knew how to get to the airport, after all. As I read through the questions on the form, I noticed the area for listing one's education. There were two lines, one for grammar school and one for high school. Something was off there. I thought lots of Ph.D.s were limo drivers! I took a hint. Nothing against driving limousines for a living, but I got the feeling I was undershooting my destiny and left without an interview.

Then one day in late August I was lolling around the garden in front of the house, bemoaning my plight. My folks' home has two extra apartments. We lived in one, and a friend from the healing school had moved in to the other. She came out to talk. I reviewed my list of financial woes with her. Then she made a comment that stuck. "I really think you've got something with your anatomy classes. At least you know what you like to do. Why don't you do something with that?" I pondered that one for a couple of weeks. I did love studying the body, and teaching. Could I really make a living just studying things I loved to learn about and then sharing that with folks who were interested to learn as well? What an exciting concept that was. I began to conjure an anatomy empire, leading throngs of somanauts into a deeper knowledge and experience of their bodies.

I didn't build an anatomy empire in a day, nor did I snap out of my depression and sense of failure on the spot, but I had begun once again to reconceive myself, and that was an important step. I have found that when it comes to reconceiving my body, how I answer the question "Who am I" is equally as important as my answer to the question "What is my body." I once read that how you describe yourself to yourself, compared over time, can prove an interesting resource for introspection and self discovery. How do you fill in the sentence, "I am _____" at any given point in your life? As a child, I saw myself as a nice person on the outside and a killer within. I never got in a fight with other kids, I told myself, because I was liable to utterly destroy my would-be opponent, much to their surprise. Such was my internal sense of grandiosity in the face of powerlessness. But controlling, holding back, and masking all of that anger and frustration took its toll on my physical form. As I've noted, by back troubles started early. In high school, I identified myself as athletic, Catholic, friendly and optimistic. I lifted weights, was heavily involved in Church youth groups, I was as nice to people as I could manage, and I had hope for the future. I no longer saw myself as nice but angry on the inside. In fact, I couldn't identify with a single emotion at all. I simply refused to feel what was going on. My weight lifting added to and cemented over the distortions in my spine, my spirituality kept me optimistic and in community, and my determination to be friendly left me in denial of how I felt about much of anything at any given time.

By the time I got to college, I moved into a whole new phase. I realized I had grown up in a home which, notwithstanding my parents sincere love and effort, was distorted by the impact of alcoholism. Denial runs deep, and I was simply incapable of grasping the impact of my circumstances until I was removed from them. For many years, I branded myself with an entirely new primary self description: I am the child of an alcoholic. Forget friendly. Now I was just pissed off. I rejected my family, blaming them for my pain and determined to stay separated from them. When I moved back home for a year after my master's degree and before beginning my Ph.D. program, the drinking was definitively a thing of the past, but I was still full of indignation regarding my family. I didn't make a very charming houseguest. It is amazing what parents will put up with from their children, even while continuing to give to them. Children throughout history have put up with their fair share as well, it is true, but grudges have a way of disabling the one who holds them first. Refusal to accept and honor one's parents "as is" will insidiously deform other seemingly unrelated relationships as well. Even marriages can break down for failure to work through grudges held by a spouse against a parent, and relationships with children of grudge-holders will suffer as well.

While I stayed there, I attended Al-Anon and ACOA meetings (adult children of alcoholics) for the year. While those meetings definitely reinforced my sense of identity as a child of an alcoholic, they did so with a major twist to my indignant version of it. At those meetings, I learned and believed that while I might be "an adult child of an alcoholic," what misery there was to be associated with that identity sprung from *my own* distorted behavior, and not anyone else's. The theme of self-responsibility ran strong through those meetings, and I slowly took it to heart. There was no room there for blaming someone else for my problems. I began to learn what a prison I had created for myself.

By refusing to take full responsibility for myself, my own character, and my own anger, I had twisted my body into a pattern of chronic pain, for which I had the audacity to blame my body. What had *I* to do with it? I also negated the possibility of having a resoundingly different experience of myself. If I play the victim, where is my power? If I place responsibility for myself outside of myself, where is my freedom? Freedom and responsibility are two sides of the same coin. Responsibility implies the power of choice. If I perceive no choice, or only one "choice," then I experience tyranny, not freedom. When I am able to recognize and acknowledge my choices, conscious or unconscious, and accept responsibility for them, to that extent I am free, free to choose otherwise, and then to act accordingly.

Identifying myself as a "victim" of my childhood circumstances, what "power" I had, if you can call it that, derived from the illusion of holding the moral high-ground. By playing the victim, I could identify with innocence, sanctity, rectitude, and moral superiority. I could identify with Jesus crucified, and all the saints and martyrs after him. I could also provoke sympathy from others: "Oh, you poor thing, how difficult that must have been!" By getting others to collude with me, to agree that I was in fact a victim of my past, I could derive outside confirmation of my plight. And there really is no shortage of "friendly and helpful" people out there willing to reinforce the identity and powerlessness of the victim. For every victim, someone is lining up to play the savior, and the two dance together. A dynamic duo, they fight some perpetrator, someone who could be blamed. Whether it be the victim's body, a disease process, "bad luck," or some "really" bad person: a boss, a spouse, a parent or relative, or some establishment authority, responsibility for "the problem" must be located outside of the victim's scope of power. Of necessity, that scope of power must be reduced to zero to maintain the role of victim indefinitely, and saviors help to confirm this, often taking responsibility for any potential or actual recovery. I traded through all of these roles, though I liked least being the one who does "wrong," as I detailed earlier. I much preferred to play the victim or savior. At least then I was posturing "in the right."

The cardinal sin in this scheme, by the way, is "blaming the victim." The stakes are high for maintaining the victim's "innocence." In the religious formulation, salvation itself could be on the line. Any hint of personal responsibility for the circumstances which the victim experiences meets with righteous indignation. "How dare you blame the victim!" From the view of the victim or the savior, "responsibility" is actually a bad thing. "Responsible" means "at fault/the cause of the problem," and "the problem" is judged as a bad thing without question. Simple logic seems to prove that responsibility is bad. The victim avoids responsibility like the plague. But that's exactly how I, by playing the victim, prolong my own suffering.

Now why, we might ask, would anyone in their right mind want consciously or unconsciously to prolong their own suffering? Well, I never claimed I was in my right mind, nor is anyone else who plays this game. But there are reasons. First, as mentioned, the role of the victim is roundly associated with innocence and holiness. And if suffering, pain, innocence, salvation, powerlessness, goodness, and righteousness are pitted against freedom, responsibility, badness, pleasure, judgment and condemnation, well, you just might believe "the suffering team" is the one to stick with, and abandon freedom on the spot. I sure did, for quite a while. Lock me up and throw away the key. However, the needling truth of the matter is, when I play the role of the victim, deep inside a part of me knows the opposite: I am truly *not* a victim, I am responsible for myself. Knowing at some level that I am living a lie, I feel guilty, and the guilty find their own punishment, one way or another. That is a second reason why someone might want to prolong their suffering. I punish myself for pretending to be a victim while "knowing" myself to be a "perpetrator." The whole set-up is pretty distorted. The guilt is actually misplaced. Guilt and judgment are essential to the logic of the victim-savior-perpetrator model, but they only "make sense" to that model. Knowing that I am responsible is no cause for guilt. Accepting responsibility is the high road to freedom. Guilt is just wallowing in the mud. Guilt feelings are merely *pretenders* to the throne of responsibility. That's why guilty people don't actually change their behavior. Guilt would vanish instantly if responsibility were truly taken up, because at that point the conscience would be clear and ready for new action.

Playing the victim, I didn't just have the company of religious folks to collude with in perpetuating the victim-savior-perpetrator drama. Not at all. Just look around and see the drama played out all around you. Read a newspaper, watch the news, go to a church, a hospital, a courtroom, listen to a political speech. People are stumbling over each other in the mad scramble to be identified as a victim, make their suffering known, and create as much distance as possible from their compelling but misplaced sense of guilt. Politicians win elections and "leaders" gain loyal and raucous followings by assuring their various victim-constituencies that their voice will be heard. African Americans are victims of white supremacy, white supremacists are victims of multi-cultural ignorance, the handicapped are victims of architectural exclusion, the obese are victims of insulin insufficiency and thyroid dysfunction, while the slim are victims of cultural programming and media indoctrination. Criminals are victims of failed socialization, women are victims of patriarchal domination, white Anglo-Saxon protestant patriarchs are victims of affirmative action policies and their domineering alcoholic patriarchal fathers who conceived them in their own image. The alcoholics, smokers and drug users are victims of advertising or addiction, and we are all ultimately victims of our "unalterable" genetic endowment, class, race, gender, sex and creed. I once even attended a meeting of bi-sexual students and watched it quickly devolve into a chorus of self-pity and victim-identification for not having been invited to the gay and lesbian club meeting. The participants were white, educated to the most elite standards, healthy and wealthy in broad measure, yet the attraction to align with the excluded and suffering victim seemed almost inexorable.

While I feel this model of the victim-savior-perpetrator is ubiquitous, and my exposure to it was deeply rooted in religious tradition, it is perhaps nowhere more heartily exemplified than in our established allopathic medical tradition and science. One of my oldest friends, my high school weightlifting chum, opted for late entry into medical school after spending some years in other fields. He had gone to Haiti, as I had, the year following my trip. While he was there, the seed was planted to become a doctor some day, and now he is a first year intern. The marathon work shifts and the relentlessly challenging process of mastering the practice of internal medicine are difficult in their own right. But, what seems to wear on him more than anything is having people place responsibility for their own or their relative's health squarely on his shoulders. He is asked to play the savior, while the sick one is the victim and the illness, body, dysfunction or "germ" is the perpetrator, baring the "blame." Doctor, patient, and disease. Savior, victim, enemy. Unless of course *he* fails to "make grandma better." In that case he *may* remain the good savior, if he clearly "tried everything possible." But he may as likely be knocked from his pedestal and vilified for *not* doing "everything possible," or worse yet, sued. Grandma didn't make it and we're calling our lawyer. Saviors are a dime a dozen, after all. They may readily be demoted to perpetrators. But victims must never be "blamed." That would pull the curtain back on the whole charade, exposing the guilt feelings of the victim, however misplaced, and their underlying sense that punishment is in fact deserved. While the rules of victim-savior-perpetrator model demand that "responsibility" be equated with blameworthiness and guilt, outside that model, we know that "it ain't necessarily so."

The demonization of the perpetrator is intrinsic to the established practice of medicine, where ancient fears of invasion and the "foreign" are played upon, once again externalizing guilt. Enemy pathogens or Germs, like Hitler's army, lurk on every front, poised for attack. Look under the kitchen or bathroom sink at the array of chemicals designed to annihilate any living thing. We buy them because it is an outstanding feature of our medical mythology to shudder at the thought of invisible dangers: bacteria, viruses, Others. I sometimes stop and wonder how our species ever made it to the 21st century, what with all those prior millennia of inept butt-wiping, rare meat chomping and unkempt cave-kitchens. From birth the medical profession engages in the desperate process of "shoring up" the body's purportedly weak and vulnerable "defense system." Pediatricians immunize infants (guilty of original immune incompetence) with the same unshakeable conviction that priests baptize the newborn (guilty of original sin). Childhood disease and original sin are vanquished with the prick of a needle or a splash from the fountain, from a universally earnest desire to serve the best interests of the children. Disease, whether physical or spiritual, is held at bay. Innocence is recovered. Fear is momentarily assuaged. At least until the kid gets measles *anyway*, or she's old enough to sin on purpose and needs to get forgiven all over again.

Despite my friends resistance to assuming the role of savior and the inherently unreasonable demands which follow, he recognizes himself to be bucking the trend. The expectation is actually assumed by both sides, the lay public and the medical profession together. They need and reinforce each other's roles. Victims need saviors, saviors need victims, and both need enemies. It may be tiring to resist being made a savior, responsible for the resolution of someone else's woes. However, it can be downright self-destructive to actually believe the myth true, and assume yourself responsible for someone else's state of health. Yet that, stunningly, is our "standard of care." Malpractice lawyers can bank on the impossibility of the standard, and juries are ready to punish. I say this not to absolve medical practitioners of their actual and vitally important responsibilities. Partnering with the sick for the betterment of health is a profound vocation and a realizable goal. Just as surely is the vocation of priest vitally important, cooperating with a community in travelling a path to wholeness and divine life. On the other hand, playing out the roles of victim, savior or perpetrator is more of a trap than a path.

So-called complementary and alternative health care practitioners are no less likely to fall into these roles as mainstream medical practitioners, despite seemingly different approaches. The roots of the problem go deeper than any particular creed or profession. I learned this slowly as a Rolfer. I had assumed that the clients I would attract in that profession would be highly self-motivated, wanting change for themselves and ready to work for it. While several indeed were, the larger percentage just wanted me to fix their aching back, foot, neck, butt or whatever. I also fell into the trap of struggling to overcome their resistance to change, as if my trying harder could somehow overcome that resistance for them. Actually, it just gave them reason to hold on more tightly, and wore me out. Despite all of my cheerleading efforts to point out how the particular ways they stood, sat, and related to people all day had a lot to do with generating the discomfort they wanted me to relieve, my clients weren't very different from me. I also would gladly have paid someone to fix me, and spare me of responsibility for my condition. While it was easy for me to fall into the role of savior as a Rolfer, like for my doctor friend, I eventually found it to be more onerous than satisfying, despite occasionally seeming to have "fixed" someone to their satisfaction. I began taking bigger chances with my clients, risking the loss of their business over playing the game, and saying things which folks might not necessarily want to hear. My time in the healing school had brought me a long way in my own ability to hear things about myself which, however painful in the moment, served my growth in the long run. I thought I would try it out in my practice. Clearly my days as a practicing Rolfer were numbered.

Along these lines, one new client in particular came ostensibly for help with his back, which he had injured in a slip-and-fall on the ice of someone else's steps. After a couple of sessions it was clear to me that his back problems had much earlier origins in his own patterns, notwithstanding the aggravation caused by the accident. However, he seemed more concerned for me to verify the depths of his injury than help him recover. He repeatedly asked if surgery would be necessary. As it turns out, he was suing the homeowners and, consciously or unconsciously, seemed to be out fishing for professional verification of his misery which would be admissible in court. I did not oblige. Instead, I told him to be careful, because the need to prove oneself a victim in court in the future could undermine his motivation to take responsibility for his full recovery in the present. After all, what jury would pity the plight of a robust and active man? I refused to support him in his role as victim, and not surprisingly, he never did come for another appointment. He needed a kind of help I was slowly learning I didn't want to give.

The history of my own case made it clear to me that the victim-savior-perpetrator model had its limitations, to say the least. For all the support and confirmations I gathered for my own chosen identity as victim-child, it sure didn't make me happy. I was separated from my family, and to that extent separated from myself, not to mention being at perceived odds with my body as well. The *illusion* of the moral high-ground to which I had crawled was a poor place to establish a real and convincing sense of moral rectitude, not to mention bodily or spiritual "health." After all, physically, I was racked with pain. Emotionally, I was racked with guilt. I used to say that "Guil't" was short for "Gilbert." I am Guilty. Now there's a cheerful identity. The internal conflict of identifying with holiness and sanctity while wanting to throttle "the people I love" was indeed profoundly guilt-provoking. Physical pain is a predictable upshot of emotional pain, I am convinced. My religious piety which supported me in identifying with the victim and the powerless also left plenty of room for acknowledging my shame and guilt and internal loathsomeness. On the bright side, a life of suffering quietly as a rage-filled victim (occasionally posing as savior) and ritually confessing one's ample guilt on a regular basis will, theoretically at least, have its rewards in heavenly bliss. My current suspicion is that "saints" of the variety into which I tried to mold myself in the past don't actually enjoy heaven either, so expertly have they mastered misery. Heaven for such is just a place to perfect one's skills as a martyr. Once again we return to the late great Bob Marley's refrain, "You think you're in heaven, but you're living in hell. Oh, time will tell, yeah, time will tell."

CHAPTER TEN

The Whole of Who I Am

The year with my relentlessly generous parents, combined with the year in the twelve step programs and their mantra of self responsibility, knocked several teeth loose in my grimacing victim identity (everyone had thought I was smiling). As recounted earlier, it took a tyrannical upbraiding from my housemate at the Rolf Institute to effect a nearly complete cure some years later. Between the two periods, I filled the growing space in my identity-gap as a Tai Chi guy, an Ex-Priest-Wannabe, Someone's Boyfriend, and an Academic. My spiritual readings and esoteric explorations into matters of the body and psychic realms altered my vision of myself profoundly. I began to formulate new ideas altogether about who I am.

For one thing, I came to believe that I am more than the personality which gets me through the day, however jolly or irritable. After all, I was developing the growing ability to step back and observe the working dynamics of my personality. To see myself from an increasingly compassionate observer's viewpoint, accept the status of my situation, and generate constructive criticism seemed to confirm there was more to me than my everyday self. Furthermore, my readings were replete with notions of reincarnation. I had been exposed to the idea in a high school anthropology class, and more heavily during my college studies. Now it became more than an intellectual curiosity. As I made efforts to see the workings of my personality, I began to view my life as a series of patterns which kept repeating with slightly different spins on them.

My relationships with people, whether family, friends, teachers, or romantic partnerships appeared to me as "works in progress" which I had been attending to for a long time, and which I would continue to reiterate until they evolved into something else. Gil's "Groundhog Day." My travels and studies felt as much a review of the past as a new experience. When I walked through Assisi in Italy where St. Francis had lived, or nearby the University of Paris in France where St. Thomas had taught, I felt like I was visiting places I had been before, and I felt as comfortable there as on any street I've lived in this lifetime.

As I engaged in scientific explorations of the body I found pointers to a larger understanding of who I am as well. I learned of the incredible constant exchange of matter in the human body. Our skin at any time is only two to five weeks old. We constantly slough off our skins like subtle snakes as the underlying tissue emerges to replace the surface cells. Those dust bunnies tumbling under the couch represent the garment of our body which we continually shed. And this is true not only for the skin, but for all the molecules which together compose our bodies. Our fat cells, our blood, the linings and substance of our organs, our very bones are replenished with new molecular content in a constant ebb and flow. It is as if our bodies are a wave winding around a river-bend rock. Whenever you look, the wave is there, but the water which passes through it is only there for the moment. The materials which compose our body flow through us like water through the wave form, ever changing. Within a year, nearly our entire body is fully renewed, and within seven, even the heaviest elements have been completely refreshed (except for those darned mercury-amalgam tooth-fillings).

So who am I? Am I the wave form through which my body flows? In a literal sense this process represents our unacknowledged ability to "reincarnate" repeatedly within this very lifetime. I am Gil Hedley for thirty-six years running, but any photo album or baby picture confirms for me that I have shed and grown quite a few bodies to represent my personality to the world. I take on different body costumes to represent my current self-conception, whether that be Baby Gilbert, Gil the Body Builder, Gil the Future Priest of America, Gil the Victim, Gil the Tai Chi guy, Gil the Rolfer, Gil the Husband, the Daddy, the Author. It seems as if my body has been a passing representation in time and space of the story I am telling about myself lately, sort of a hard-copy holo-gram of my personality. And if my personality is capable of gener-ating body after body over the course of my human life span, it does not seem to me so great a leap to conceive that my spirit, ever conscious and perceptive of my doings, is capable of generating personality after personality over the course of many human life-spans. And as surely as my body has seemingly followed the growth of my evolving personality, perhaps my personalities over time are proceeding in a course of growth following the evolution of my spirit. There is a general quality or character to who I am, which I feel is ever so slowly curing, mellowing, and ripening. Eventually there may come a time to pour me out of the bottle for good, but for now at least I am still maturing in the vintner's care.

With my exposure to Daskolos, that late Greek Orthodox healer from Cyprus I mentioned earlier, I pressed the question "Who am I?" even further. Daskolos, or Stylianos Ateshlis by name, was keen to emphasize the "I am" of who I am. In the story from the He-brew Torah, when Moses stood before the burning bush, Moses asks "If the people ask for the name of the God who sent me, what shall I say?" God replies to Moses, "I AM WHO I AM. Tell the people of Israel I AM (YHWH) has sent me to you." Clearly God is not caught up with personality-level issues here. As Daskolos notes, among ourselves, one says "I am George," another "I am Helen." The personal name follows the divine name for all of us, and the question is, with which one do we choose to identify more strongly: with "the petty time and place personality," or with the divine life and Spirit which animates every one of us as a shared source. If I say "I am Gil," where is my emphasis, on "Gil" or on "I am?" Is there room for both in my self-conception? When I say "I am Gil," and remember that scripture passage, it's a pleasant surprise and reminder for me that Gil and the Divine Name are uttered in the same breath. As it says in the Koran, "Allah is as close as your jugular vein." Exploring who I am at this level, the divine life and Spirit appears as the common thread which is woven through us all. When I awake in the morning and re-assemble "Gil" for a new day, knowing "Who I am" makes all the difference. I am in good company.

Karen and I both took this transformation of our self-conception to heart. Our healing school placed great emphasis, as did Daskolos, on this recognition and openness to accept the manifestation of the divine life within us. The ethical implications are profound. How will I care for myself if I acknowledge the divine presence forming who I am? How will I treat my neighbor, spouse, child, parent, sibling, stranger, student, friend or "enemy" if I am willing to acknowledge the divine presence inherent in them? Saying "I am _____" carried both weight and power, and we took it seriously. At a particular point in the ritual of the Roman Catholic mass, upon viewing the consecrated bread and wine, the congregation together states "Lord, *I am not worthy* to receive you, but only say the word, and I shall be healed." We found that we could no longer speak those words with conviction. "*I am worthy*" seemed to us a much more powerful truth to pronounce than "I am not worthy." What worthiness I possess derives from the truth of who I am, not the pretension of who I am not. If the divine life animates my very being, how dare I deny my worthiness? Only my "petty time and place personality," posing as my victim-self, would deliberately choose to split off from my divine source and proclaim my "unworthiness."

For a while, we just switched the words and mumbled them differently amid the general proclamation. We belonged in New Jersey to a generally progressive congregation and we very much enjoyed both the community and our involvement in it. For quite a while we had simply adjusted our participation here and there to accommodate for our shifting beliefs and identities. My Catholic identity had run strong through me my whole life. But eventually we adjusted our participation right out the door. The ritual repetition of my sinfulness, my unworthiness, my low place on the church-hierarchical totem pole on a weekly, if not daily basis, had always been sufficiently resolved in the past for me with the "punch-line" that I was nevertheless forgivable and saved: I shall be healed. But now I was hearing those same words which I had been repeating all of my life, and the punch-line didn't overcome my increasing sense of self-betrayal for having spoken them. How shall I ever be healed if I keep splitting myself off from my divine life and my body, separating myself from myself? I did not deny my numerous faults and failings, I simply tired of paying them greater due than they deserved. I stopped identifying with them as the crux of who I am. I wanted to focus my attention on the truth of the divine light shining within me, rather than reiterating and identifying with my petty failures. Judge not. I began to quiet the voice of self-judgment. I began to stop wallowing in guilt. These are long-term projects. I have not rooted out all of the places in my life where I betray myself habitually. I am conscious of the task, however.

Our "stepping out" of our church community was sealed for us when we decided to baptize Sarah ourselves. We had struggled for months about baptizing her into the Catholic Church. Notwithstanding our sincere love for that community, our willingness to raise her in the ritual forms and structures of the Church and to create in her that particular identity had atrophied severely. The contemporary Catholic baptismal ceremony, filled with powerful symbolism and meaning, really is more about welcoming a new person into the community than it is about "washing away original sin," though that is definitely still part of the package. We balked at having Sarah welcomed into a community we were in the process of leaving. Instead, we invited family and friends to our backyard, where we ceremonially dunked Sarah Grace Hedley into the deep brook which ran through it. Karen and I wanted to hold a ceremony of "identification" for our daughter, along the lines of Jesus' baptism. When Jesus was baptized by John in the river Jordan, the Holy Spirit is said to have descended upon him like a dove, while a voice from heaven proclaimed "This is my beloved son, in whom I take delight!" Standing hip-deep in a trout stream with Karen, dipping and drawing from the water our na-ked soaking ten-month-old wriggling like a fresh catch, we hoisted her aloft and proclaimed the same, "You are our beloved daughter, in whom we take delight." With crayfish nibbling at our toes, we knew the joy which parents find in their children, as the "divine parent" did in Jesus. Sarah can safely say that "God knows who I am, and my folks do too."

Coming to a different sense of who I am, a broader, fuller, more integrated sense, also enabled me to begin to reconceive my body in a way that I could not from my victim-identity. As I have implied, the answers to the questions "Who am I?" and "What is my body?" are intimately related. It is nearly impossible as a vic-tim to reconceive my body. Reconceiving my body implies a choice for a different experience, but as a victim I don't like having choices, so I am stuck with my body as is. Choice goes back to that respon-sibility issue, and I can't be a victim and be responsible simulta-neously. Whether I am a religious or medical science style victim, I experience my body as separate from myself, and posing a threat. My body, like the foreign pathogens which invade it, is a problem to me, gives me pain, hurts me. My body is responsible, not me. The body alienated from the self assumes the role of the enemy. As a religious victim alienated from my body, it becomes legitimate to deprive my body or otherwise torment it in an effort to bring it in line or conquer it. Spirit and body are split, and opposed. Spirit is over the body, ruling the body. The mind, or reason, is often set aside in religious formulations, or it can be seen masquerading as spirit, demanding its way. On the medical science model, it is considered fair play to silence my body through "symptom relief," inject my body with lethal chemicals, blast it with radiation, or literally carve pieces of it away in order to "save the patient." Mind and body are split, and opposed. The mind rules over the body as in a hierarchy: the brain is king, the body, serfdom. If the peasants are revolting, starve, torture and defeat them. Here the spirit is set aside as fanciful nonsense, the domain of the churchman. The machine is spiritless. The body is reputed to be in the wrong on either model. If it "acts up," it is a problem, it is responsible, it is judged, and it is punished.

The good news is that the time and place identities which I choose pass on like fall leaves, which dry up and blow away. New ones eventually grow. If "I am a whole person," for instance, then my body becomes integral to who I am, and not separate from me. It is an aspect of my personal expression for which I am in large measure responsible. And if I stress the "I am" in the identity "I am a whole person," then I must respect all of me as bearing the divine life: body, mind and spirit. In that case, no aspect of me as a person can rightly be betrayed or rejected. I must accept the whole package to experience my integration fully. My scientific mind cannot reject the prodding of my spirit; admitting to spirit will not render the mind inconsequential or displace true knowledge or reason; and placing my body in a circle of communication with mind and spirit rather than subjugating it to one or the other will only enrich the whole. Acceptance is the counterpoint to judgment here. Spirit, mind and body each have significant contributions to make to the whole, and each deserve to be given full voice. As St. Paul wrote, can the hand say to the foot, I don't need you!?

Yet how many times has my mind, bent on pursuing some goal at work or play, shut-up the voice of my body? My body will first whisper its needs: I'm thirsty, I'm hungry, I'm tired, I can't support that weight safely, I need a better chair, Put on a jacket, Go for a walk, Get some fresh air, some sunshine, some pleasure. My body speaks to me through the language of sensations, which I may choose to feel or ignore. If I do choose to ignore the initial subtle messages of sensation, my body will increase the volume and grab my attention with more acute sensations of pain. Now *I am in pain* (as opposed to *my body is killing me*). If I ignore those shouts of my body still, I risk injury, disease, even physical death. My body may begin to speak in the language of more extreme sensations, systems may shut down, or parts may be split off from the whole and operate "as if they had a mind of their own."

To the mind habitually self-patterned to rebut, reject or ignore body sensations, it may actually seem as if the body in fact has nothing to say. "I feel fine" should here be translated "I feel nothing," or, more accurately, "I refuse to feel anything." It's as if the mind can relegate sensation to the deep freeze. I know that one from personal experience. I eventually had to accept that feeling was possible for me, and that refusal to feel was an habitual choice which I could change. Reconceiving myself as a whole person, I reconceived my body as well. I could begin to see how feelings of pain were not personal attacks from my alien body or punishments from God indicting me for real or imagined moral wrongs, but important internal communications of myself to myself which deserved my attention. Yet from my victim-perspective, the voice of my body met with my judgment and condemnation. Pain was bad, a problem to be fixed. Problems were bad, implying I was somehow "wrong." I thought I had to defend myself.

Shifting to the whole person perspective, there is no room for judgment of my body and its language: its voice is my own. I require no defense. My body is the current physical form of my self. Shutting it up is self-betrayal. If I attend to what my body has to say for the whole person that I am, and accept the pain or problem I am experiencing as an extremely accurate sensory representation of where I am in the moment, I open up new possibilities for myself which my judgments had excluded. When I meet my body's voice with judgment, I split myself. "I" judge "it" before "it" judges "me." I struggle to maintain my innocence, and stand as a victim of my body, in pain, sick. I assume a place where there is no power to change or choose differently, settling for the illusion that I may be under attack from the "outside," but at least I am "right" and "blameless." When I meet my body's voice with acceptance, I can experience my whole self, which may be characterized by some imbalance at the moment or even habitually. But I do not sacrifice my "innocence" by taking responsibility for being in pain here. My body finds no "fault" in me, nor does my spirit. My "innocence" is never even at stake in this model. That's the victim's worry. I simply notice and create the possibility for another choice. As a whole person, responsibility represents the path of freedom to choose a more fulfilling experience, given my recognition that my current choice is not so satisfying. The language which my body speaks to the whole contains not a whit of judgment. Bodily sensations are what they are. They arise from within as signals of the character of my experience in a given moment. As a whole person, I can monitor my experience through bodily sensations and make choices based on that information. On this scheme, judgment, blame, splitting off from and silencing the voice of the body have no place at all. They belong to a different story which I have told about myself to myself. That story frankly bores me now, because I told it for so long, and never improved my situation for having done so. Life as a whole person is a lot less stressful than life as a victim. I feel better. My spirit whispers who I am, my body senses the truth of it, and with my mind I choose what to do with it all. Looking back, I can understand why I experienced more integration lying there wiggling on the floor at that Continuum workshop, enjoying a few moments of self-generated pleasure in my back, than I did in all my years of struggle to fix my body. In creating that experience for myself, I recognized through stark counterpoint that I actually did have a choice regarding how I experienced my physical self. My spirit lay waiting like a mirror in my heart of pleasure. In accepting responsibility for the choices I had made in the past, I empowered myself to enjoy other options.

A whole person, I also found, is not an isolated identity. While as a victim I shared my world with saviors and perpetrators, and other victims, and endured the isolation of pervasive guilt and defensiveness, as a whole person I found a larger world to enjoy. Experiencing my "internal" connections enabled me to experience the larger fabric of my world more fully. Connecting to my love for my family more than to my grocery list of their offenses, real or imagined, I was able to create a relationship with Karen that previously was beyond the practical limits of my self-conception. Relinquishing my judgment of my family, simply letting it go, I became less critical of myself, and so less likely to criticize Karen. Not feeling judged herself, I didn't provoke so many negative reactions in Karen as I had in past relationships, and we both felt safe to be open to each other's love. "Good measure, pressed down, shaken together, running over, will be put into the fold of your garment, because the measure that you measure out will be measured back to you." No judgment there. Just simple, straightforward math. Opening myself to love provoked a sense of and desire for even more connection, within and without. An entirely different feedback loop was begun.

So I got a lot of mileage out of shifting my sense of who I am. And by reconceiving my body as a current physical expression of who I am, I saw the incredible connections within my body itself as a "local" demonstration of my pervasive interrelationship with the surrounding world and beyond. As surely as no divisible "part" of my body exists in isolation from my whole body or my whole self, no identifiable "whole person" exists in isolation from the greater universe. I am connected. I am one. We can create models which reduce reality to a series of isolated parts, but the illusion of separation can never definitively supplant the fabric of connections, despite our choices to act according to a model rather than the larger reality.

As surely as I had found support in our society at large, in my religious background, and in the culture of science and medicine for upholding my victim identity and separated body, I found I could mine the depths of those same general resources and find support for myself reconceived as a whole person. In science, I discovered a whole "sub-culture" of thought had developed in the shadows for the last hundred and fifty years. "New" Biology, Holistic Physics, Sacred Geometry, "Alternative Medicine" and others had already understood much of what I was only beginning to discover. Since the time of Pasteur and the development of the

germ theory, other less popularly acclaimed but not less meaningful voices sought to focus our attention within. Instead of whipping up fear of "invading pathogens," these research scientists held
to the belief that to maintain my health I need to take responsibility for the "internal milieu" or "terrain" of my body. For these
folks, "invasion of a pathogen" was a symptom of an internal imbalance which left the door open to a disturbance. The solution,
therefore, was not to kill off the invader indiscriminately and at
any cost, but to support and restore internal balance, and so render the internal milieu of the body inhospitable to the "invaders."

The research of these scientists supported their view that the
healthy, balanced human body is host to a great many cooperating
little microbial creatures, symbionts. Our normal functioning de-
pends on these microbial symbionts, who live within us and enable our bodily life. On a good day, we provide them with safe
harbor, and they help with our life processes. The fact is, bacteria
and other life forms inhabiting our body, cell for cell, outnumber
our mammalian cells by a hundred to one. Literally trillions of life
forms teem within us. Our healthy bodies are thriving, coopera-
tive communities. Digestion and nutrient assimilation (some argue even cell division) are dependent upon help from these symbionts. However, if my body's internal milieu becomes inhospitable to these cooperating organisms, they will move into stages of
their life cycle which enable them to survive in the shifted environment.

Many things over which I exercise control may create such a
shift in my body's internal environment. Chronic poor diet, lack
of exercise, shallow breathing, impure water, poor air quality and
insufficient sunlight: all of these can sour my body over time. Anxiety, held emotional stress, anger, hostility and chronically poor
personal relationships can also measurably distort the internal chemistry of my body. Negative emotions actually generate a toxic internal milieu. Happiness is a definitively healthier condition. Furthermore, many medicines themselves, designed to alleviate symptoms, may alone or in combination so distort my body's internal

balance that even more medicines are "needed" to alleviate new symptoms arising from the initial intervention. Overuse of antibiotics wipes out friendly as well as "unfriendly" bacterial populations, as well as selecting out strains of new and heartier "perpetrators." That can lead to further internal imbalance. When our normally friendly symbionts are sufficiently provoked into their survival mode by these imbalances, we may perceive their changed forms (or the external company which they now attract) as an invasion, an infection, a growth or tumor, or some other disease state. Relative to us, they stop functioning as symbionts and start functioning as pathogens.

At this point, apart from recognizing the role we play in generating these circumstances, we are liable to see the disease as the main problem. We will enlist help for our plight, and often engage the most complex solutions to vanquish the symptoms, when the deeper roots of the problem are in fact simple, general, and overarching. I, for instance, thought I needed to understand the intricacies of spinal mechanics and the details of spinal musculature to "outsmart" my back and overcome my chronic pain. Actually, I needed to give myself permission to choose pleasure for myself more often. By doing so, I created much more powerful positive shifts in the internal milieu of my upper back than any amount of well meaning surgery or bodywork would likely have accomplished. While the choice may seem naively simple at face value, the story of my life so far shows at the very least that I have generated innumerable "reasons" and obstacles to make that choice seem a poor one, and unworthy to be made.

In fact, I must admit that with my exposure to the alternative science I actually fed my anger for a while. Like with the vaccination issue already discussed, I would vent about establishment medical science crushing its opponents like a church crushing heretics. I would actually poison my internal milieu with my anger even while talking about self-responsibility for maintaining it in a healthy state. The irony was not lost on one of my anatomy students from the healing school, who was also a classmate and friend.

She approached me one evening after class, and gently pointed out that if I continued to present these issues in such a hostile way, not only would I fail in the long run to convey my message and its importance, but I'd probably make myself sick as well, if there was any truth at all to the theories. I remain indebted to her comments, which snapped me back into focus once again. Reading about people whose books had been burned by government authorities, who had been vilified by the medical establishment, tried on spurious charges and even jailed for promoting their beliefs, I stirred my own fear bubbling within, and reacted with anger. I ranted to Karen and my students, I wrote letters to congress, testified at hearings, got a lawyer, gathered information, and learned "my rights." But taking my friend's comments to heart, I remembered I could take a different tactic altogether. If I am a whole person, with the divine life pulsing in me, what did I really have to fear? Running with fear, I would invariably revert to my angry, split, obsessive, posturing, innocent victim-identity, full of judgment and righteous indignation (all the while fearing I might actually have done something wrong). When I remembered who I am, and aligned myself as a whole person, I could actually detach from those fears and talk about the same issues with compassion and humor. When I am a whole person, and I am remembering the same of others, I can see past the play of victims and perpetrators going on all around me and know I have nothing to fear. What a relief. I still revert frequently enough to my victim identity, but at least I know I have options.

I also found ample religious resources to support a growing sense of who I am as a whole person. Among them, the teachings of Daskolos revealed for me an esoteric side of Christianity that bypassed the victim-savior-perpetrator drama in favor of the path of theosis, discovering and identifying with the divine life within. Daskolos embraced the study and development of one's body and appreciated the spectacular intelligence and resource it represents. He expected the research of truth to happen at every level, and feared nothing from the insights of science. For him, the road of the opening mind was the likelier path to wholeness than dogmatism. Perceiving science to be in its infancy still, he would argue that there is properly no metaphysics, but only physics partially understood. We have a lot to learn, and need never mask ignorance with fear or fantasy. Now get to work!

Scripture has always been a favorite resource for me as well, and I have exposed myself to the sacred writings of numerous religious traditions. One thing seems certain. I am capable of interpreting every tradition to support my most painful choices as well as my most fulfilling ones. Steeped in the Christian tradition more than any other, I had no trouble identifying with the victim-perpetrator-savior model as I saw it spelled out in the New Testament. Short of writing another book on the matter, I will say I have returned to the same texts with a renewed identity and sense of my body and found vastly different insights and meanings waiting there for me. In the past, I was attracted to Jesus' command to "take up your cross and follow me" and "place my yoke upon your shoulders." I reveled in the idea of suffering with Jesus, like old pals in martyrdom. Returning to the passage with the knowledge that I am a whole person, I find myself more apt to ponder what follows: "For my yoke is easy and my burden light." I had never wanted to hear that part, I guess. Easy. Light. I can live with that now. And can I, by focusing on Paul's universal identification that "all men are sinners," have much time to reflect on Jesus' declaration, "I am the light of the world," coupled with his equally compelling statement to his listeners that "you are the light of the world." If Jesus says he is the light of the world and I am the light of the world, then I think I will busy myself moving mountains with faith, and greater things even still, rather than waste my time wallowing about in guilt, supposedly grateful for my savior, and busy pointing out to anyone who can stand to listen that, by the way, you are all sinners too. A reconceived identity transforms perception and behavior. A reconceived body transforms experience and its meaning.

CHAPTER ELEVEN

Moving On

Karen, Sarah and I eventually welcomed Christopher Gabriel into the world three days before Christmas, 1997. If Sarah's essential character is sweetness, his is joy. He was born on the very same spot in the very same hot tub, but this time Karen noticed that the unseen crowd of Native Americans who showed up for Sarah's birth were displaced by old crones and midwives, invisibly coaching Karen along with our midwife. Christopher's birth had a certain fierce swiftness to it: he was "out" within two hours of labor's onset. With Sarah in my mother's arms watching, and me in the tub with Karen, she delivered him "in the cowl," birth membranes intact. It was at sunrise when I fished my son from the waters, and he's been the first one up every morning since! A truly robust little fellow, we named him on Christmas, after the day itself and the angel who announced it. It was the best Christmas of my life. I really felt a member of my holy family.

We grew out of our little three room basement rental apartment on the spot, though it took another year and a half for us to move. Meanwhile, we encroached severely on my parents' space, taking over a couple more rooms of their house for work and play. They were thrilled to have their grandchildren born and growing under their roof, and accommodated us while Karen and I plotted our move. At this point, neither of us was Rolfing anymore. She was a mother of two, and I had grown my "anatomy empire" to the point where we were living from my teaching income alone. I continued to offer weekend classes and workshops in Manhattan.

A friend who started a healing school in western Pennsylvania invited me to teach her groups as well. I had also expanded the number of my dissection workshops, creating opportunities for folks to study "integral anatomy" with me in other cities across the country. I began to advertise nationally, and between that, word of mouth, and mailing tons of postcards, I actually created a fulltime business based on my excitement for exploring the "inner space" of human form. I became a "somanaut" in my own right.

Just a few months ago, we reached the point where I could relinquish my local weekend teaching commitments on the east coast. For years we had wanted to move west and raise our kids in the foothills of the Rocky Mountains, where Karen first doodled my fingers (!). We rented a house with more then twice the room we'd been using. It feels like we have literally taken the lid off of our lives as we look up at the huge expanse of sky stretching out over the great plains. The sky really is the limit. I remain deeply committed to the process of incarnation. Along the lines of that project, I devoted myself to writing this book as the first of a series in which I explore the theme of reconceiving our bodies. To be perfectly honest, what I wrote over the last ten chapters surprised me. I had set my intention to write on the theme of "reconceiving the body" in general in this first volume, and quickly realized that I needed and wanted to speak for myself, from my heart, rather than maintaining the kind of dispassionate distance which earned me my Ph.D. My head can be a lonely place. I wanted to find company with the reader and myself in my heart. I plan for the next volume of this series to be titled *Reconceiving Our Bodies, Volume II: Integral Anatomy*. I want to share in that book the more particular understandings of our shared human form which I have developed while teaching anatomy over these past six years. I am looking forward to writing that one as much as I have enjoyed committing the preceding to paper.

Beyond writing, I have additional aspirations for the growth of my "anatomy empire." I have recently incorporated The Creative Research Institute and Learning Center, LLC. I am still actively studying and employing the principle of leverage to develop, fund and implement this project fully. I plan to expand on the research which I have begun on my own and with my classes. I also want to showcase and advance upon the accomplishments of research scientists for whom I believe the world in now ready. At the Creative Research Institute and Learning Center, I want to explore with both the young and the grown the nature of human form, the whole person, and the relationships of the larger whole. I want to do this in a way that includes the insights which can be derived from body, mind and spirit working in partnership with the intelligence of nature and the divine life which animates all creation. The overarching purpose of the Creative Research Institute and Learning Center is to foster personal and planetary integration and healing through these explorations. At this point, the project is newly conceived. To quote Sarah, "I'm *so* excited!"

Thanks for reading along. I truly appreciate your interest.

Printed in the USA
CPSIA information can be obtained
at www.ICGtesting.com
CBHW030807230624
10283CB00003B/7

9 780738 818214